*Psychology Revivals*

# Selective Mutism

Originally published in 1981, this title was designed to present a comprehensive review of research on, and treatment of selective mutism. It represents the only systematic overview of research and treatment procedures on this behavioral problem at the time. In many respects the literature on selective mutism clearly presents the differences in assessment and treatment between the intrapsychic (or psychodynamic) and behavioral approaches to deviant behaviour. The title presents an overview of the two major therapeutic approaches of human behaviour within the context of treating selective mutism.

# Selective Mutism
## Implications for research and treatment

## Thomas Kratochwill

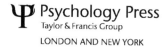

Psychology Press
Taylor & Francis Group

LONDON AND NEW YORK

First published in 1981
by Lawrence Erlbaum Associates, Inc.

This edition first published in 2014 by Psychology Press
27 Church Road, Hove, BN3 2FA

and by Psychology Press
711 Third Avenue, New York, NY 10017

*Psychology Press is an imprint of the Taylor & Francis Group, an informa business*

**Publisher's Note**
The publisher has gone to great lengths to ensure the quality of this reprint but points
out that some imperfections in the original copies may be apparent.

**Disclaimer**
The publisher has made every effort to trace copyright holders and welcomes
correspondence from those they have been unable to contact.

A Library of Congress record exists under ISBN: 0898590647

ISBN: 978-1-138-84957-0 (hbk)
ISBN: 978-1-315-72502-4 (ebk)
ISBN: 978-1-138-85008-8 (pbk)

# SELECTIVE MUTISM:
# Implications for
# Research and Treatment

Thomas R. Kratochwill
*University of Arizona*

**LEA**

LAWRENCE ERLBAUM ASSOCIATES, PUBLISHERS

1981    Hillsdale, New Jersey

Lawrence Erlbaum Associates, Inc., Publishers
365 Broadway
Hillsdale, New Jersey 07642

**Library of Congress Cataloging in Publication Data**

Kratochwill, Thomas R
  Selective mutism.

  Bibliography: p.
  Includes indexes.
  1.  Mutism, Elective.  I.  Title.  [DNLM:  1.  Child
behavior disorders.  2.  Mutism—In infancy and childhood.  WM475 K895s]
RJ506.M87K72        618.92'855        80-18631
ISBN 0-89859-064-7

Printed in the United States of America

To Carol Ann, Tyler Thomas, and
my parents, Marian and Rudy

# Contents

# Preface

My work as a practicing psychologist and as a university professor responsible for training psychologists has exposed me to a variety of childhood behavior disorders. Several years ago, I observed cases in which children had zero or near-zero frequency of speech in select settings. Careful analysis of these cases suggested that the children not only spoke in select settings or with certain individuals (e.g., parents), but also that they had relatively normal or intact speech in other respects. This set them apart from children who experienced severe retardation, language disorders, autism, or severe psychotic disturbances.

Exposure to these mute children prompted my colleagues and I to search the relevant clinical literature for various therapeutic procedures that would assist in the development of effective intervention programs. Of course, many behavioral treatment strategies for speech- and language-disordered children as well as for adult mute psychotics were readily available. However, we also found that a rather sizable literature existed on what was commonly labeled ''elective'' or ''selective'' mutism. Much of this literature, particularly the early cases reported, came from the intrapsychic or dynamic model of deviant behavior. The behavior therapy literature on childhood mutism, also sizable, has rapidly grown in the past few years and provided many excellent treatment examples.

At that time, it became apparent that there was no systematic review of the literature on selective mutism. The prospect of contributing a review to the behavioral literature was exciting. Discussing problems with research and treatment of a particular behavioral problem within the context of contemporary research methodology in behavior therapy was even more exciting. After reviewing the intrapsychic and behavioral literature in the area of childhood mutism, and after finding useful treatment procedures as well as methodological problems in each area, I decided to undertake the present volume.

The book is designed to present a comprehensive review of research on, and treatment of, selective mutism. The book represents the only comprehensive overview of research and treatment procedures on this behavioral problem. It extends some of the earlier work published by the author and his associates (Kratochwill, Brody, & Piersel, 1979), wherein a select portion of the intrapsychic and behavioral approaches to therapy are reviewed. It also extends the work of Sanok and Ascione (1979) in which behavioral interventions were reviewed and evaluated. In many respects the literature on selective mutism clearly presents the differences in assessment and treatment between the intrapsychic (or psychodynamic) and behavioral approachs to deviant behavior. The present volume presents an overview of the two major therapeutic approaches of human behavior within the context of treating selective mutism.

The research methodology within the intrapsychic and behavioral approachs offers dramatic contrasts in objectivity and replicability. It will be obvious to the reader that while behavior therapists have far outdistanced their intrapsychically oriented colleagues when it comes to research methodology and description of useful therapeutic procedures in some cases, much work remains to be done in both areas. The methodology of behavior therapy has been actively evolving and is becoming a sophisticated technology for measuring clinical behavior change. Both of these features are reflected in the methodological review of the childhood mutism literature presented herein. Specifically, a methodological critique of the childhood mutism literature is presented to elucidate future research and treatment strategies in this area.

The literature reporting treatment of selective mutism suggests involvement by such fields as education, school and clinical psychology, social work, psychiatry, and speech. The present volume will be useful for individuals conducting research in this area as well as for practitioners seeking treatment plans for mute children. My ultimate hope is that individuals from diverse fields will extend research on childhood mutism as well as employ some of the recommended treatment strategies described herein to improve the adjustment of these children.

Many people contributed to this work. I was most fortunate to have the comments of Benjamin B. Lahey on the manuscript. The development of this manuscript was also supported by my wife, Carol Anne, and my son Tyler, who remained mute during certain periods of my writing. My special appreciation goes to my parents Rudy and Marian who assisted in editorial work on the manuscript. Many thanks are also extended to Naomi Van Gilder and Judy Landrum for their extensive work on the project. Finally, I wish to thank Larry Erlbaum and the staff at Lawrence Erlbaum Associates for their efforts and support of the work.

# SELECTIVE MUTISM:
## Implications for
## Research and Treatment

# 1

# Selective Mutism: Issues in Diagnosis and Classification

Anyone who has been engaged in treating children's behavior disorders will appreciate the diversity of influences that are related to maladaptive functioning. Deviant behavior during childhood represents a composite of environmental, genetic, and social-cultural influences. With such potential diverse influences, it is no wonder that there are literally thousands of books dealing with different aspects and perspectives on normal and abnormal functioning in children. Certain theoretical and philosophical perspectives on human functioning largely determine specific definitions of deviant behavior, as well as normative standards, and ultimately influence how such problems are treated.

Presented in this book is an examination of different approaches to the research and treatment of children commonly labeled "electively" or "selectively" mute. Salient characteristics of this population of children and the active processes in treatment and research that result in labeling them as deviant are discussed, as well as methods for improving this process. Methods of treatment and research are discussed from two different approaches that reflect the predominant orientations of published studies involved with treating childhood selective mutism. These approaches include the intrapsychic, or psychodynamic, and behavior modification, or behavior therapy, models of human functioning. Because the intrapsychic and behavioral models represent different conceptual and methodological approaches to deviant behavior, both approaches present sometimes diverse assessment and treatment strategies.

In this volume, the term *behavior modification* and *behavior therapy* are used synonymously. Although some writers have attempted to distinguish the terms, contemporary arguments suggest that there has been no consistent usage, and generally there is little to be gained by making distinctions (see Kazdin &

Wilson, 1978; Wilson, 1978). My approach in the present volume is primarily behavioral in that recommendations for future treatment and research are based on behavioral procedures. Some of the characteristics of the behavioral approach toward assessment and treatment are detailed in Chapter 3. The interested reader should also consult several primary sources for an extensive overview of behavior modification (e.g., Bandura, 1969; Kazdin, 1975, 1978a; Kazdin & Wilson, 1978; O'Leary & Wilson, 1975; Ross, 1974; Sulzer-Azaroff & Mayer, 1977).

Before embarking on an overview of the intrapsychic and behavioral appraoches to treatment and research on selective mutism, some issues relevant to diagnosis and classification are presented. Of necessity, this involves a brief overview of some of the major issues raised in diagnosis and classification of behavior disorders. The present discussion is not intended to be comprehensive, for this would involve a major work in its own right. Indeed, there have recently been major texts devoted to the topic of psychiatric diagnosis (Rakoff, Stancer, & Kedward, 1977; Spitzer & Klein, 1978), and chapters and journal articles have proliferated. The interested reader is referred to these sources as well as to several major publications that provide a detailed discussion of this area (Adams, Doster, & Calhoun, 1977; Begelman, 1976; Cromwell, Blashfield, & Strauss, 1975; Phillips, Draguns, & Bartlett, 1975; Quay, 1979; Ullmann & Krasner, 1969).

## DIAGNOSIS AND CLASSIFICATION

Throughout the history of psychology and psychiatry, individuals have endeavored to differentiate various types of behavior disorders and to describe their unique features. An important step in the study of behavior, and particularly deviant behavior such as mutism, involves grouping observations into an organized scheme. Classification has provided a process of identification of phenomena, so that events may be measured and communicated among professionals. In medicine, the search for disease entities proved valuable because advances made in diagnosis were related directly to treatment and specific understanding of etiology. Unfortunately, at this time, psychology and psychiatry have failed to provide a comprehensive system of classification that unifies and transcends specialty areas (cf. Adams et al., 1977).

Over the past 100 years, various mental health professionals have been engaged in description, treatment, and research on a child behavior disorder that is characterized in its behavioral manifestations by a lack of functional speech in all but a few select situations and/or with certain individuals. Both intrapsychic and behavioral researchers have tended to *label* the problem in similar ways. That is, both groups have tended to use a common term to describe this problem. This might be regarded as a major problem for the behavioral approach, which typically has not held labels and traditional diagnosis in high regard. For example,

Phillips et al (1975) were critical of the behavior modification approach for using conventional classification schemes. They suggest that behavior modification has not yet succeeded in completely eschewing classifying entities. They further point to the fact that some behavior modification texts (e.g., Ullmann & Krasner, 1969; Yates, 1970) still divide the subject matter into chapters corresponding to traditional diagnostic units. It might be added that this is true of many recent texts examining various aspects of behavioral treatment and assessments (e.g., Hersen & Bellack, 1976; Kazdin & Wilson, 1978). Of course, the focus of this book is on a deviant behavior that has been labeled ''elective'' or ''selective mutism,'' and so such a criticism might apply here as well.

However, the argument against behavior therapists for their use of conventional classification schemes is not substantive. Defining a particular behavior disorder is a hazardous task, particularly when one considers the field of abnormal psychology and the problems that have accompanied diagnosis. Indeed, the very task of defining is complex and multifaceted. Begelman (1976) suggested that there are at least 11 distinguishable activities in the clinical literature that have been identified as defining: namely, categorizing, stipulating, substituting, abstracting, disturbing, operationalizing, verifying, mapping, theorizing, judging, and pointing.

In the case of mutism, stipulatory definitions have been a common form of defining this problem used by behavioral researchers. Stipulatory definitions involve a speech convention. Thus, with regard to the problem of mutism,

TABLE 1.1
The Various Terms Used to Describe Children Who Speak Only
in Select Settings and/or Only to Certain Individuals

| Label | Author(s) |
|---|---|
| 1. Elective mutism | Elson, Pearson, Jones, & Schumacher, 1965; Wulbert, Nyman, Snow, & Owen, 1973 |
| 2. Functional mutism | Amman, 1958 |
| 3. Reluctant speech | Williamson, Sewell, Sanders, Haney, & White, 1977b |
| 4. Selective mutism | Kass, Gillman, Mattis, Klugman, & Jacobson, 1967; Kratochwill, Brody, & Piersel, 1979; Piersel & Kratochwill, in press |
| 5. Speech avoidance | Lerea & Ward, 1965 |
| 6. Speech inhibition | Treuper, 1897 |
| 7. Speech phobia | Mora, Devault, & Schopler, 1962 |
| 8. Speech shyness | Nadoleczng, 1926; Rothe, 1928; Spieler, 1941 |
| 9. Suppressed speech | Sanok & Striefel, 1979 |
| 10. Thymogenic mutism | Waternik & Vedder, 1936 |
| 11. Voluntary mutism | Kussmaul, 1885 |
| 12. Hearing mute | Adams, 1970 |
| 13. Temporary mutism | Kanner, 1975 |
| 14. Negatism | Bakwin & Bakwin, 1972; Rigby, 1929 |

various writers have established, through convention, that the term *elective* or *selective mutism* will be used as the name (label) for a particular pattern of behavior. Of course, one problem with this approach is that different researchers have used quite different labels to refer to the same or similar behavioral patterns. Whereas Tramer (1934) is commonly credited with lauching the term *elective mutism* in the clinical literature, the German physician Kussmal described "voluntary" mutism in association with insanity as early as 1877 (cf. Von Misch, 1952). But these are only a few of the terms that have been used to describe a pattern of behavior in which a child does not speak in certain situations and/or to certain people. Table 1.1 shows the various *labels* that have been used to describe this behavior pattern. Nevertheless, the vast majority of these terms deviate little from Tramer's (1934) original portrayal, in which the *behavioral manifestation* was exhibiting abnormally silent behavior outside all but a small group of intimate relatives or peers.

The point is that both behavioral and intrapsychic writers have used similar terms, but the approach toward assessment, diagnosis, and treatment differ markedly between the two. This is best reflected in a brief overview of the two contrasting approaches to diagnosis of deviant behavior in general.

## Traditional Diagnosis

A traditional view of mental disorder has been conceptualized within medical concepts of the nature of illness. Within this framework, the individual exhibiting disturbed or deviant behavior is considered sick and is suffering from an illness that prevents normal adjustment to society (Phillips et al., 1975). The medical model has expanded in recent years (Spitzer & Klein, 1978). One of the major problems with past attempts to classify deviant behavior is that a disease model from medicine has been applied to behavior. The application of a disease model (either in its literal or metaphorical sense) to abnormal psychological behavior has led to attempts to identify specific disease entities or processes. In the case of its literal application, seven or more decades of biological, biomedical, and genetic research have isolated remarkably few physical bases for recognized forms of psychopathology (Phillips et al., 1975). Of course, the application of the medical model to physical disease remains one of the most remarkable features of contemporary science.

When used in its metaphorical sense (as in psychoanalysis, where symptoms are considered an expression of a clash among incompatible processes within the personality that can be traced to early childhood experiences), it has not fared well either. Present-day diagnostic schemes can be traced to the German psychiatrist Emil Kraepelin (1856-1926), who developed a diagnostic system that exerted a major influence on psychiatry (cf. Kazdin, 1978a). The major features of Kraepelin's system and his basic approach toward mental deviance have been largely retained. The past, current, and future editions of the *Diagnostic and Statistical Manual of Mental Disorders* (DSM-I, DSM-II, and DSM-III [see

American Psychiatric Association, 1968, for DSM II] demonstrate their Kraepelinian heritage, as do many textbooks in abnormal psychology (e.g., Cole, 1970; Coleman & Broen, 1972; London & Rosenhan, 1969; Suinn, 1970; Ullmann & Krasner, 1969) and psychiatry (e.g., Arieti, 1959; Freedman & Kaplan, 1967; Mayer-Gross, Slater, & Roth, 1969). Spitzer and Endicott (1978) make the cogent point that classifications of mental and other medical disorders have existed for decades despite the lack of any agreed-on definition of what constitutes a medical disorder in the first place. Even official classification schemes of the World Health Organization (The International Classification of Diseases) and the American Psychiatric Association (the first and second editions of DSM) made no attempt to address the issue.[1] Although a dissatisfaction with DSM-II has led to the development of DSM-III, the new DSM reflects a close affiliation with the medical model and has retained many of the problems of DSM-II (cf. Schacht & Nathan, 1977).

What is involved in the new American Psychiatric Association's *Diagnostic and Statistical Manual of Mental Disorders* (third edition), or DSM-III? The DSM-III is undergoing field trials and by the end of 1981 will likely be in general use.[2] Generally, DSM-III provides for the diagnosis of mental, medical, and psychosocial conditions presented by clients within several diagnostic "axes." A number of recent works have reviewed various issues in the conception and use of DSM-III (cf. McReynolds, 1978; Quay, 1972; Schacht & Nathan, 1977; Spitzer, Sheehy, & Endicott, 1977; Spitzer & Williams, 1980; Zubin, 1978). The DSM-III adheres to a multiaxial diagnostic system in which five axes will be referenced in diagnosis of an individual—namely: (1) clinical psychiatric syndromes and other conditions; (2) personality disorders (adults) and specific developmental disorders (children and adolescents); (3) nonmental medical disorders; (4) severity of psychosocial stresses; and (5) highest level of adaptive functioning in the past year (McLemore & Benjamin, 1979). In the area of mental disorders (axes I and II), there are over 230 separate categories of disturbance, representing a 60% increase in the total number of psychiatric disorders contained in DSM-II and a 280% increase over DSM-I (McReynolds, 1978).

Like its predecessors, DSM-III adheres to a categorical, disease-entity conception of behavioral disturbance. Spitzer et al. (1977) defend this position:

> The justification for using a categorical approach in DSM-III which treats psychiatric conditions as separate entities connotating entity status if not denoting it lies in the practical utility of such topology for communication, treatment, and research,

---

[1]For a brief overview of DSM-II, DSM-III, the World Health Organization (WHO) system, the International Classification of Diseases (ICD-9), the system developed by the Group for the Advancement of Psychiatry (GAP), and the California I-Level system, the reader is referred to Quay (1979).

[2]For further information, see the following report: American Psychiatric Association, *Task Force on Nomenclature and Statistics, DSM-III draft.* Available from Robert L. Spitzer, M.D., 722 West 168th Street, New York, New York 10032.

> despite theoretical limitations. Furthermore, the history of medicine attests to the value of categorical subdivision in the discovery of specific etiology and treatment [p. 6].

Thus, we have a new DSM that is based on the medical model and that describes many new instances of "psychiatric" disturbance.

Over the past few years, a considerable amount of debate has occurred in the area of diagnosis and the use of traditional classification schemes, especially DSM-I and II. Begelman (1976, pp. 23–24) summarized nine somewhat overlapping criticisms of the DSM system. One has been added to his list (see 10). Generally, the problems can be summarized from several perspectives (cf. Adams et al., 1977; Begelman, 1976; Hersen, 1976; Marholin & Bijou, 1978; McLemore & Benjamin, 1979; Phillips & Draguns, 1971; Rhodes & Paul, 1978; Spitzer & Klein, 1978; Spitzer & Wilson, 1975): (1) excessive reliance on the medical model of abnormal behavior (e.g., Adams, 1964; Albee, 1968; Begelman, 1971; McReynolds, 1978; Szasz, 1960; Ullmann & Krasner, 1969); (2) facilitating the stigmatization of individuals (e.g., Farina & Ring, 1965; Goffman, 1973; Laing, 1967; Millon & Millon, 1974; Rosenthal & Jacobsen, 1968; Sarbin & Mancuso, 1970; Scheff, 1973; Stuart, 1970); (3) employing debatable theoretical notions (e.g., Cautela & Upper, 1973; Panzetta, 1974); (4) poor or low reliability and validity (e.g., Barlow, 1977; Salzinger, 1978; Sandifer, Pettus, & Quade, 1964; Schmidt & Fonda, 1956; Seeman, 1953; Stoller & Geertsma, 1963; Zubin, 1967); (5) little relevance toward prognosis, treatment, and future prediction of behavior (e.g., Adams et al., 1977; Derschowitz, 1974; Goldfried & Kent, 1972; Hersen & Barlow, 1976; Mischel, 1968); (6) dehumanizing the client–therapist relationship (e.g., Laing, 1967); (7) poor consistency of categorical groupings (e.g., Cautela & Upper, 1973); (8) promoting biases that stem from arbitrary decision rules (e.g., Millon, 1969; Panzetta, 1974); (9) promoting a perception of homogeneity among individuals labeled the same (e.g., King, 1951; Wittenborn, 1951, 1952; Zigler & Phillips, 1961a, 1961b); and (10) the erroneous extension of adult disorder labels (schizophrenia) to child problems (e.g., childhood schizophrenia; e.g., Eisenberg, 1969; Phillips et al., 1975).

Perhaps one of the best indications of the utility of traditional diagnostic schemes is addressing how well they have worked in the past. In a review of research studies that were concerned with certain aspects of psychiatric diagnosis, Franks (1969) concluded:

> The review of this research leaves one with the uncomfortable feeling that the results of all the studies that have utilized psychiatric diagnosis as a dependent or independent variable are of questionable validity. The data reviewed herein suggest that an entirely new system of classification is needed, one which can encompass the many variables that define psychological functioning and behavior in the hu-

man, including the viewing of these functions from a developmental frame of reference [p. 167].

A similar conclusion was reached in a subsequent review (cf. Franks, 1965) and by others who have called into question the relevance of traditional diagnosis for treatment (e.g., Bannister, Salmon, & Leiberman, 1964; Carson, 1969).

Generally, the reliability of the DSM-II system remains largely uninvestigated (Quay, 1979). For example, in a study measuring the utilization of the categories of DSM-II in a single clinic, Cerreto and Tuma (1977) noted that their results must be tempered by the unknown reliability of various assigned diagnostic labels. Although there was some evidence that some of the diagnoses listed in the DSM-II were being applied more infrequently (cf. Phillips et al., 1975), it appears that the development of DSM-III will lead to more frequent usage as well as to past problems that have characterized DSM-I and DSM-II. Some criticisms of DSM-III have already emerged, with the most salient limitation noted as its adherence to the traditional medical model. McReynolds (1979) noted:

> The medical model is no longer heuristic in social science. What good it brought to our discipline was exhausted long ago. It now entraps our thinking and limits our research and practice. This is true not only for the disease entity conception of behavioral processes but for all categorical representations of behavior, be they mental disorders, personality types, or other notions of behavioral discontinuity. In sum, there is little reason to expect a decade of new research on DSM-III to produce findings that substantiate the categorical approach to understanding and modifying unwanted or troublesome behavior. That well is dry [p. 125].

Other recent criticisms follow many of those advanced against DSM-II. Three listed by McLemore and Benjamin (1979, p. 18) are noteworthy. First, diagnosis still rests partly on impressionistic clinical judgment (e.g., global ratings of the severity of psychosocial stresses and of the patients' highest level of adaptive functioning during the past year). Indeed, the DSM-II, DSM-III, WHO multi-axial system, the ICD-9, GAP, and California I-Level System all represent clinically derived classification systems all sharing problems of reliability and validity (Quay, 1979; Zubin, 1967). Second, the DSM-III system categorizes individuals in terms of illness very broadly defined. Third, DSM-III shows a near total neglect of social psychological variables and interpersonal behavior. More-over, it appears that despite the real and potential advances in scope, diagnostic reliability, and diagnostic logic of DMS-III, it remains a potentially poor document and may be bad for psychologists[3] (Schacht & Nathan, 1977).

---

[3]The new DSM-III may be bad for psychologists for political reasons. Its professional and legal significance for psychology appears troublesome, because promulgation of DSM-III as an official action of the American Psychiatric Association will carry sufficient weight to call it to the attention of insurers and legislators, who will perceive it as quasi-official recognition of the primacy of physicians in the diagnosis and treatment of the disorders categorized therein (See Schacht & Nathan, 1977, for a more detailed discussion of DSM-III).

## Traditional Classification of Childhood Mutism

The field of child psychopathology is typically faced with an even greater challenge in classification of behavior disorders than are individuals attempting to establish adult classification schemes (Phillips & Draguns, 1971). As Phillips et al. (1975) have noted: "To an even greater extent than with adults, classification of psychopathology in children is based on externally judged social transgressions or deficiencies in intellectual or social performance [p. 41]." Childhood behavior problems are sometimes closely interwoven with normal development and should be analyzed within the context of the expectations of both therapist and responsible socialization agents.

Within the traditional intrapsychic approach to childhood mutism, one finds a variety of terms used to describe this problem (see Table 1.1). An individual operating from the intrapsychic orientation and employing DSM-II had a number of options to labeling the mute child. For example, one might use the "Transient Situational Disturbances" (307.1 adjustment reaction of childhood) or a category that is reserved for more stable, internalized, and resistant to treatment than *Transient Situational Disturbances,* such as "withdrawing reaction of childhood" or "overanxious reaction of childhood" or an "other" category. Laybourne (1979) suggests that in the DSM-II, mutism is "withdrawing reaction of childhood 308.0" and in the GAP, the syndrome is properly designated as "overly inhibited personality, elective mutism." Of course, the diagnosis typically would be made on the basis of the total performance of the child rather than the mutism per se. Within the ICD-9 system, elective mutism would be classified as "Disturbance of Emotions Specific to Childhood and Adolescence," usually characterized with anxiety and fearfulness. Within DSM-III, elective mutism (313.23) is classified as "other disorders of infancy, childhood, or adolescence."

What diagnostic issues have been raised in the intrapsychic literature? A variety of perspectives have been suggested. Browne, Wilson, and Laybourne (1963), cited a report by Glanzman in which mutism was tied to an "anal sulker syndrome", in which the three main symptoms were total or elective mutism, urinary retention, and voluntary retention of stools. Nadoleczng (1926) indicated that the electively mute child may have a "weak speech impulse" or be "speech shy." Whereas Treidel (1894) observed that the cause of mutism was in factors that constituted the symbolic content of language (i.e., it was easier for such children to imitate words than to speak voluntarily), Gutzmann (1912) noted that mutism occurred in children with a speech defect and most typically occurred after being teased by peers. None of these early accounts was based on extensive empirical data.

Waternik and Vedder (1936) offered classifications of childhood mutism based primarily on precipitating factors rather than symptomatic manifestations. Spieler (1941) referred to four varieties or types of mutism (i.e., hysterical, elective, thymogenic, ideogenic) resulting from psychogenic causes. In the hysterical variety, the child was said to speak in an emergency, thereby simulating partial "elective mutism." Later, Spieler (1944) reviewed 50 cases of mutism and suggested that neurotic personality was the outstanding feature of mute children.

As is true of many childhood disorders, early writers defined mutism somewhat by exclusion (e.g., Morris, 1953; Tramer, 1934). Tramer (1934) distinguished selective mutism from language retardation, schizophrenic mutism, and other forms of mutism but included hysterical reactions. Some writers perceived mutism as being closely tied to other forms of intrapsychic personality patterns. Weber (1950) stressed a specific disposition to reactions of stupor and depression in mute children. Noteworthy was the supposed abnormal dependence on the mother, which was hypothesized to relate to oral dependency needs and was but a form of regression to early infantile social relations. Heuger and Morgenstern (1927) related a case of childhood mutism in which partial mutism developed into total mutism. In concert with Freudian theory, the authors reported that the child continued to communicate through drawings, and they proposed that the disorder was caused by castration anxiety.

Von Misch (1952) and Weber (1950) reported cases of selective mutism that presented similar histories and etiologies. The families of these children were reported to be very withdrawn (e.g., little social contact in the community) and demonstrated signs of neurotic and psychotic disorders. The children were also described as low in intellectual ability and poorly adjusted to strangers. Von Misch (1952) observed: (1) Environmental factors may precipitate mutism; (2) mutism often occurred upon the child's separation from the family (e.g., upon entry into school); (3) the disorder was primarily psychogenic, although heredity and intelligence have a role; (4) all cases demonstrated excessive ties to the mother; and (5) selective mutism was possibly related to a traumatic experience at the time speech was developing.

Different classifications of selective mutism have developed, with some authors considering it a neurotic reaction (e.g., Elson, Pearson, Jones, & Schumacher, 1965) and others labeling it a personality trait disturbance (e.g., Pustrom & Speers, 1964). Halpern, Hammond, and Cohen (1971, p. 95) presented a variety of conditions that characterize or cause mutism: (1) a predisposing constitutional hypersensitivity to instinctual drives (as manifested by social reticence), (2) traumatic events experienced during critical periods of language development (as in teasing speech attempts), (3) an insecure environment (as in child abuse); (4) a psychological fixation (as in utilizing mutism as a fear-reduction mechanism); (5) a neurotic symptom that represents a compromise arising out of familial conflicts involving talking, openness, and dependency; and (6) an association with such problems as school phobia, speech defects, obstinacy, enuresis, withdrawal, compulsivity, and separation difficulties.

Halpern et al. (1971) offered a formulation of selective mutism similar to that presented by Leventhal and Sills (1964) in their discussion of school phobia. Halpern et al. (1971) note:

We understand the mutism as a speech phobia arising out of an overevaluation by the child of his power. The own voice, perceived as faulty or weak, becomes inferentially invested with the potential power when it is held desperately in abeyance. Therefore, it is not so much the power of speech as the power of silence or retention with which the affected child controls an unfamiliar world. His success in evading verbal transactions with the nonfamilial people in his environment can only further strengthen omnipotent fantasies of being "the strong, silent type [p. 97]."

Laybourne (1979) distinguishes between primarily elective mutism and secondary forms of the disorder. Whereas children who manifest elective mutism characteristically refuse to speak in school and to strangers (but who do speak to specific people), secondary forms of the disorder occur in which failure to speak is part of the "symptomatology." This occurs in cases of hearing loss, schizophrenia, hysterical aphonia, and aphasia. Other writers suggest that mutism, but not necessarily selective mutism, occurs in childhood schizophrenia and early infantile autism (e.g., Kanner, 1975; Shirley, 1963). Bakwin and Bakwin (1972) note that the basis for elective mutism is usually family pathology. Rutter and Hersov (1977) note that whereas elective mutism is usually a "pure" emotional disorder, mutism may develop as a reaction to an underlying speech or language handicap. Thus, some children avoid speech because of the teasing and mockery they receive for mispronunciation or other speech defects. In a rather extensive discussion of "mutism among psychotic children," Etemad and Szurek (1973) note that in their review of 264 psychotic children seen in the Langley Porter Neuropsychiatric Institute Children's Service between 1946 and 1961, 80—or 30%—were totally mute or showed a marked paucity of verbal expression relative to expected age norms.

Finally, Kaplan and Escoll (1973) have described a form of "adolescent elective mutism" that has its onset after the age of 12 years. They present two

TABLE 1.2
Comparison of Childhood and Adolescent Elective Mutism[a]

|  | Childhood Elective Mutism | Adolescent Elective Mutism |
|---|---|---|
| Onset | Before age 6 | After age 12 |
| Partial mutism | With peers, strangers, therapists | With family and therapist |
| Chief complaint | Does not talk | Stealing, conversion reactor, suicide attempts |
| Dynamics | Preoedipal | Preoedipal, oedipal genitality |

[a]After Kaplan and Escoll (1973).

case histories of adolescent females who had not spoken to their families for 1 to 3 years prior to treatment. Table 1.2 presents their contrast between the child and adolescent forms of mutism. The authors noted that the major dynamics of the two girls were separation, a prohibition against the expression of anger from adolescent to parent, and a sexually stimulating relationship between the girl and her father. Specific discussion of this case occurs in Chapter 3 of this volume.

There are, of course, other characterizations that could be offered from the intrapsychic literature. Generally, writers from this orientation share a concern for the appropriate description of internal dynamics to explain the selective mutism. In yet another body of literature, an analysis of environmental contingencies and a focus on actual behavior are used to describe mute behavior.

## Behavioral Diagnosis

The behavioral approach to diagnosis generally represents a contrast to the intrapsychic model. Numerous authors have demonstrated the lack of a functional fit between conventional diagnostic categories and various behavior modification techniques (e.g., Franks, 1969; Kanfer & Saslow, 1965; Ullmann & Krasner, 1969; Yates, 1970). In contrast to the intrapsychic model, in the behavioral approach it is not considered necessary to understand underlying dynamics to change behavior. Thus, behavioral diagnosis focuses upon specific target behaviors and the conditions under which they are performed. Although individuals affiliated with a behavioral approach may use labels to discuss an area (e.g., elective or selective mutism, social withdrawal, school phobia), behavioral diagnosis is generally not aimed at assigning individuals to traditional diagnostic categories. In this regard, diagnosis is aimed directly at assessment for purposes of developing a treatment program.

Yet some behavioral writers have noted that the avoidance of diagnosis or classification has hindered the development of behavioral assessment strategies (cf. Ciminero & Drabman, 1977). They note that behavior therapists have not been arguing against diagnosis (or classification) per se, but rather have criticized the actual methods used to gather data, the types of data collected, and the interpretations of those data in terms of underlying causes of behavior (see also Salzinger, 1978). In the words of Achenbach (1974), ''The basic question is not *whether* to classify, but *how* to classify [p. 543].'' Nevertheless, the already developed classification systems (as represented by the GAP [1966] and DSM-I, II, and III) have been rejected, mainly on grounds already discussed.

Over the years, several conceptual diagnostic schemes have been proposed in the behavioral literature. One of the early descriptions of behavioral diagnosis was provided by Kanfer and Saslow (1965, 1969). The system is designed to improve the decision-making process about specific intervention programs. The system consists of seven steps (Kanfer & Saslow, 1969):

> 1. An initial analysis of the problem situation in which behaviors brought to the attention of the therapists are sorted out with regard to their eventual place in

treatment. Target problems are sorted into (a) behavioral excess (i.e., in terms of frequency, intensity, duration, and occurrence under conditions when a behavior's socially sanctioned frequency approaches zero), (b) deficients (e.g., responses that fail to occur with sufficient frequency, adequate intensity, appropriate form, or under socially expected conditions), and (c) behavioral assets (e.g., nonproblematic behaviors).

2. A *clarification of the problem situation* that examines environmental factors (e.g., stimulus conditions under which the behavior[s] occur[s], and consequences that may maintain the behavior[s]). This analysis stems from the assumption that deviant behavior requires continued support.

3. A *motivational analysis* is conducted in which both positive and aversive events are examined.

4. A *developmental analysis* is conducted in the context of (a) biological (e.g., vision, hearing), (b) sociological (e.g., SES), and (c) behavioral changes (e.g., deviance from social norms).

5. An *analysis of self-control* is conducted to determine what behavior the client can control (independently.)

6. An *analysis of social situations* is conducted to elucidate the relation of individuals in the client's environment to reinforcing or aversive qualities that may control behavior.

7. Finally, an *analysis of the social-cultural-physical environment* is conducted to examine the normative standards of behavior and the client's limitations and opportunities for support (e.g., family support) [pp. 430-437].

Kanfer and Saslow (1969) suggest that these steps have the purpose of defining a client's problem in a mannor that suggests specific treatment operations and specific behaviors as targets for modification. Although the approach can be employed as a guide for the initial collection of data, as a device for organizing data, or as a design for treatment, it is not a substitute for assignment of the client to a traditional diagnostic category. Kanfer and Saslow (1969) suggest that such labeling may be desirable for statistical, administration, or research purposes, but the behavioral diagnosis is intended to replace other diagnostic formulations purporting to serve as the basis for making decisions about specific therapeutic interventions (p. 437).

It should be noted that the Kanfer and Saslow (1969) system does not suggest how the therapist should *combine* data. Dickson (1975) noted:

While the Kanfer and Saslow (1969) format for functional analysis provides the behavior therapist with a systematic procedure for gathering data, it does not allow a scientific approach in interpreting the data collected. Thus, the behavioral assessor is still very much an artist in selecting those behaviors for intervention, in deciding what frequencies define excesses or deficits, and in discriminating whether to intervene within the environment containing the controlling stimuli, or within the organism [p. 365].

Kazdin (1978a) noted that in practice, no concrete system of behavioral diagnosis is followed. More typically, the behavior therapist discusses general classes of behavioral problems in terms of behavioral deficits, excesses, inappropriate stimulus control, and aversive response repertoires (e.g., Bandura, 1968; Bijou & Grimm, 1975; Bijou & Peterson, 1971; Bijou & Redd, 1975; Kratochwill & Bergan, 1978; Marholin & Bijou,1978).Behavioral diagnosis is closely linked to assessment and treatment. Indeed, behavioral diagnosis leads directly to treatment, because a major purpose of diagnosis is to reformulate the client's problem in behavioral terms, to define the conditions under which the behavior occurs or fails to occur, and to select a treatment strategy. As Marholin and Bijou (1978) note: "Diagnosis or assessment is, instead, oriented toward attaining the kinds of information or data that can be directly used to *develop and guide a treatment program* [p. 15]."

Realizing that some sort of classification scheme may prove useful in research and practice, the movement toward a more formal system of behavioral classification has recently been proposed (e.g., Adams et al., 1977; Cautela & Upper, 1973; McLemore & Benjamin, 1979; McReynolds, 1978). The system developed by Cautela and Upper (1973), called the Behavioral Coding System (BCS), provides general descriptive categories of maladaptive behaviors (e.g., fears, addictions, sexual disorders, thinking disorders, antisocial behavior, self-injurious behavior, and inappropriate habits of daily living). Within each category, several specific behavioral variations are enumerated to add greater flexibility and specificity (Kazdin, 1978a). Generally, the BCS is designed for cataloging problems in terms of specific, directly observable behaviors. In this regard, inferences in the behavioral diagnosis are minimized. Like the Kanfer and Saslow (1969) system of behavioral diagnosis, the BCS does not suggest what type of treatment program should be designed.

Adams et al. (1977) have chosen a method of organizing behaviors that is based on a scheme of response systems similar to the classification system used in physiology. Their system, called the Psychological Response Classification System (PRCS), unlike the DSM-II and DSM-III, classifies responses rather than people. Thus, by defining a unitary set of phenomena, the eliciting stimuli, the responses to treatment, the theoretical inferences, and so forth have been placed in the perspective of empirical questions or eventual explanatory laws. In this way, the system encourages the empirical investigation of theoretical disagreements rather than obscuring or excluding them. The authors note that the PRCS has several specific aims:

One is to take arbitrary assumptions regarding distinctions between normal and abnormal responses out of the alpha level of classification. Unless it is empirically demonstrated to be otherwise, abnormal behavior is considered to be an extension of normal behavior and similar in kind. Many difficulties have arisen from attempts to classify symptoms as distinct from nonsymptomatic behavior. It is not the proper role of an alpha level classification scheme to make value statements about what is normal and abnormal. Abnormal behavior can be defined only in the context of what is normal, which is an empirical question [p. 67].[4]

The PRCS is divided into motor, perceptual, biological, cognitive, emotional, and social response systems. Each system is accompanied by a definition, a response category, and further definition. The utility of the PRCS in clinical practice is that it: (1) gives the therapist an opportunity to test the degree of definingness of the popular data language of psychology; (2) shows that many psychological terms or concepts must be defined further so as not to obscure important diagnostic differences or produce ambiguous communications; (3) makes the presence or absence of relations among response syndromes a clinical decision based on client observation rather than theoretical assumptions; (4) provides the therapist with a model by which to organize and evaluate the usefulness of various assessment devices and treatments that are relevant to each response system (and subsystem); and (5) reflects the progress of psychology with regard to information generation pertinent to response systems (and subsystems) (Adams et al., 1977, pp. 75–76). The PRCS holds promise as a useful classification system for behavioral psychology, but much work remains to be accomplished before it becomes a completely workable system. One criticism of the PRCS is that it does not specify the clinical implications of various combinations of responses from the six categories (McLemore & Benjamin, 1979). In actuality, the system will be quite complex to employ.

Yet another approach that provides a close approximation to behavioral classification systems for children is what has been developed from a dimensional approach using multivariate statistical methods (i.e., factor analysis and cluster analysis). This approach assumes that there are a number of independent dimensions of behavior and that each individual exhibits the behavior to a greater or lesser extent (see Quay, 1972, 1979; and Ross, 1974, for an overview). Quay (1979) noted that in the building of a classification system, the statistical approach clearly obviates two of the basic weaknesses characteristic of the clinical approach. First, empirical evidence is obtained showing that a dimension exists as an observable constellation of behavior. Second, the objective nature of most of the constituent behaviors permits reliability of the measurement of the degree to which the child manifests the dimension (p. 12).

The multivariate statistical approach basically attempts to isolate clusters of behaviors that occur together. Ciminero and Drabman (1977) note that although

---

[4]The development of a classificatory system begins with the construction of lower-order categories referred to as an "alpha taxonomy" (cf. Brunner, Goodnow, & Austin, 1965). In this level of classification, the basic terminology or the operational definitions of science are constructed. The construction of an alpha taxonomy requires a thorough description of the observable attributes of phenomena within a specified set (see Brunner et al., 1965, and Adams et al., 1977, for further discussion of this issue).

it is possible to view a cluster of behaviors within a traditional conceptualization or as a syndrome of some underlying disorder (cf. Mischel, 1968), it is also possible to interpret the cluster in terms of response–response relations. Moreover, such response clusters can become a legitimate concern in behavioral assessment, with important implications for treatment (O'Leary, 1972; Wahler, 1975).

Attempts to identify clusters of child behavior problems have been made, especially with various rating scales (cf. Achenbach, 1974; Quay, 1972, 1979; Ross, 1974). Two factors have emerged from this effort with some consistency. The first factor, variously termed *conduct disorder, aggressive, unsocialized, psychopathic, or externalizing,* is viewed as excessive acting out or aggressive behavior. Teacher and parent ratings, case history data, and children's self-report data have demonstrated the existence of this "factor" in such settings as schools, clinics, and other institutions. The second factor, variously termed *overinhibited, personality disorder, withdrawn, or internalizing,* is viewed as excessive withdrawal and has been found in several settings. According to Ross (1974): "These categories differentiate excess approach behavior (aggression) and excess avoidance behavior (withdrawal) [p. 28]." Recently, Quay (1979) reviewed studies that provide characteristics defining the category "Anxiety-Withdrawal." Such children may be characterized as anxious, fearful, tense, withdrawn, reticent, and so forth. Likely, many children who would exhibit selective mutism could be classified in this category.

Nevertheless, this potential approach, though promising, does not represent a comprehensive classification system. A problem with the approach is that the frequency with which these behavior patterns are found is probably due to the sample of children studied and the type of data selected (Ciminero & Drabman, 1977). In this regard, it would be difficult to identify the behavioral deficits that might be found in, for example, a retarded population, because data from this group are frequently not included in factor analytic studies (cf. Ross, 1974). Second, much of the data gathered for the previous factor analytic studies have come from rating scales that suffer from reliability and validity problems. Moreover, the format of those scales differs considerably in item content, rating instructions, and operational specification of the behavior being rated. Although the factor analytic approach holds promise, other classification schemes (such as those described earlier and hereafter) may provide a better alternative in behavioral diagnosis and classification.

McReynolds (1979) has offered a sociobehavioral classification system of behavioral disturbance. This approach is based on the premise that individuals are identified for psychiatric care because their behavior is disturbing to themselves or others. This puts the analysis (diagnosis) within a sociopsychological conceptualization. Within this approach, one person can present a behavioral disturbance to another in two ways: (1) "the first's (person's) actions disturb the second such that it is the presence of responses or behavior patterns that is disturbing''; or (2) ''there is an absence of specific responses or response patterns, and the failure of the designated deviant to engage in certain behaviors poses the disturbance'' (McReynolds, 1979, p. 129). The format allows behavior to be classified as excess (former case) or as deficit (latter case). In this regard, the system is similar to other behavioral diagnostic systems (e.g., Kanfer & Saslow, 1969; Ross, 1974). For example, Ross (1974) provided a definition of a behavior disorder that employs a similar conceptual scheme: ''A psychological disorder is said to be present when a child emits behavior that deviates from a discretionary and relative social norm in that it occurs with a frequency or intensity that authoritative adults in the child's environment judge, under the circumstances, to be either too high or too low [p. 14].''

These two broad categories of socially defined disturbance are further described on five behavioral dimensions (i.e., frequency, duration, and magnitude, latency, and context) and by a subdivision of behavior into cognitive, affective,

TABLE 1.3
Sociobehavioral Classification of Residual Behavioral Disturbance[a]

---

I. Social conditions of residual disturbance
  A. Identity of complainant relative to designated deviant
    1. Self
    2. Family or family member
    3. Community agency
    4. Civil or criminal authority
    5. Helping professional
    6. Employer
    7. Friend
    8. Other
  B. Complainant request for designated deviant
    1. Behavior change
    2. Behavior control
    3. Partial removal
    4. Total removal
II. Behavioral nature of residual disturbance
  A. Behavioral complaint
    1. Excess
    2. Deficit
  B. Response dimension
    1. Frequency
    2. Duration
    3. Magnitude
    4. Latency
    5. Context
  C. Action system
    1. Cognitive
    2. Affective
    3. Motor
    4. Somatic

---

[a] McReynolds, 1978, 1979.

motor, and somatic actions. For example, a thought is a cognitive action; autonomic nervous system arousal is a somatic action; anger is an affective action; and speech falls into a motor action category. This classification scheme is presented in Table 1.3. The three classes and $2 \times 5 \times 4$ subclasses of disturbing behavior in the second half of the table identify 40 behavioral events that can lead to a ''complainants'' designation of someone as potentially deviant.

This system has potential because of the operational specifications that can be used with various behavior disorders. However, like the former systems, much work needs to be done to make the system empirically based.

The system proposed by McLemore and Benjamin (1979) is also based on an interpersonal behavioral approach. Generally, their approach represents a general method for translating traditional diagnostic categories into psychosocial terms. The system is based on Benjamin's (1974) work in which she used both the clinical and nonclinical literature to develop a model of social behavior called the *structural analysis of social behavior* (SASB). Space limitations preclude explication of the system and its many applications. Table 1.4 lists the criticisms of DSM advanced by Begelman (1976), along with a description by McLemore and Benjamin (1979) of how their system compares with the traditional DSM approach. Generally, a good deal of work has already gone into conceptualization and empirical analysis of the SASB. However, it too has far to go in the development of a rigorous taxonomy of social behavior.

## Behavioral Diagnosis of Mutism

Arriving at a satisfactory definition of selective mutism is primarily a methodological issue, both in assessment and in research. Whereas many psychodynamic writers have characterized mutism as part (or a symptom of) a more global personality disorder, in behavioral assessment (diagnosis) and research, an operational definition is most frequently identified as the target behavior subjected to modification. Those individuals operating from a behavioral orientation toward diagnosis and treatment have tended to define mutism as a problem in terms of frequency of talking (speech) in certain select situations and/or to certain individuals (cf. Kratochwill, Brody, & Piersel, 1979). Kratochwill et al. (1979) noted that there have been some difficulties in uniformity of definitions in various behavioral research studies. First, most behavioral researchers have relied on convention and adopted the term *elective mutism* (e.g., Richards & Siegel, 1978; Williamson, Sanders, Sewell, Haney, & White, 1977a; Wulbert, Nyman, Snow, & Owen, 1973; Yates, 1970). Based on early psychodynamic writings, such children were characterized as ''electing'' to remain silent (cf. Tramer, 1934). Although this is not a problem per se (see earlier discussion of stipulatory definitions), it does raise the issue of whether a new term might be more useful for sharing research and treatment procedures among professionals.

Second, a number of different populations have been subsumed under the umbrella term *mutism*. Behavioral procedures have, of course, been used for the

TABLE 1.4
Interpersonal Diagnosis and Criticisms of the DSM[a]

| Criticisms (from Begelman, 1976) | Comparison with Interpersonal Nosology |
|---|---|
| 1. Overreliance on the "medical model" | Interpersonal diagnosis treats reports and observations of social behavior as its units of analysis and thus in no way fosters a belief in "disease processes"; it at least implicitly suggests continuity between the normal and the abnormal, and though it does not necessitate adherence to any particular etiological theory, it easily lends itself to learning formulations of *pathogenesis* and *therapy* (what many interpersonal theorists would rather term *development* and *remediation*). |
| 2. Stigmatization of those diagnosed, especially the institutionalized | Although virtually any set of conceptual categories can be imbued with value attributes, interpersonal description is relatively free of stigmatization, whereas DSM categories seem to encourage the view that the person is his disease ("Mr. Jones is a schizophrenic"; H. E. Adams et al., 1977, p. 49); social behavioral response characteristics are not taken to be dispositional (intrinsic to the nature of the individual). |
| 3. Incorporation of debatable theoretical notions | Since all nosologies are essentially theoretical, and nearly all theoretical notions are potentially debatable, there is little to be said here except that an interpersonal nosology is eminently researchable (testable). |
| 4. Inadequate reliability and validity | Though the reliability of traditional diagnostic labels is notoriously low, we discuss elsewhere in this article the rather respectable reliability of interpersonal assessment, along with issues related to construct validation; determinations of criterion-oriented validity must be made with reference to specific contexts (e.g., how well an interpersonal taxonomy predicts responses to particular treatments). |
| 5. Little value for prognoses, specifications of treatment, or predictions of general behavior | When contrasted with the DSM, interpersonal assessment would seem strong in these domains; the interpersonal models allow for either situation-specific or generalized behavioral predictions (the validity of the former will of course be higher; cf. Mischel, 1968, 1973|c.); of perhaps even greater potential value are the clear implications for treatment specified by an interpersonal evaluation (see Dimond, Havens, & Jones, 1978, for a relevant discussion). |
| 6. Dehumanization of the therapist–client relationship | All classification systems, to the extent that they result in the objectification of the client, may be said to dehumanize the therapist–client relationship; by contrast with the DSM, however, interpersonal taxonomies do not imply any qualitative distinction (e.g., sick vs. well, ordered vs. disordered) between the client and the clinician, at least insofar as both manifest nearly all interpersonal behaviors in varying degrees. |
| 7. Inconsistencies in categorical groupings | Such inconsistencies do not arise in interpersonal taxonomies, which are explicitly constructed around internally consistent models of human behavior. |
| 8. Biases toward pathology (e.g., diagnosing in terms | Since an interpersonal nosology is not a collection of heterogeneous entities, this problem does not emerge; it could, but |

*(continued)*

TABLE 1.4 (*continued*)

| Criticisms<br>(from Begelman, 1976) | Comparison with<br>Interpersonal Nosology |
|---|---|
| of the most "severe" behaviors evident in cases of "mixed symptomatology") | need not, arise when the interpersonal diagnostician is comparing an individual's responses to, say, a friend or employer (which may be relatively functional) with those to a spouse or parent (which may be relatively dysfunctional). |
| 9. Presumptions of homogeneity among individuals similarly labeled | Diagnostic labels will probably always function somewhat as stereotypes (H. E. Adams et al., 1977, p. 54), and therefore the presumption of homogeneity within categories is perhaps inescapable; the crucial issue becomes how narrow or broad to make nosological categories (or dimensions); interpersonal taxonomies have the highly desirable property of flexibility on what Cronbach (1970, pp. 179-182) has called the "bandwidth-fidelity" dimension, the trade-off between breadth of coverage and precision of measurement—Consider the molecularity of the Benjamin model versus the relative molarity of the Leary circle; consider also that the former may be collapsed into a small number of quadrants. |

[a] McLemore & Benjamin, 1979.

treatment of numerous speech problems, including autistic mutism (e.g., Wolf, Risley, & Mees, 1964) and childhood schizophrenic mutism (e.g., Isaacs, Thomas, & Goldiamond,1960). Although the vast majority of children are labeled electively mute (or another suitable term—e.g., selectively mute), some children have been labeled elective mute when demonstrating little functional speech across all situations (e.g., Blake & Moss, 1967). It seems reasonable to categorize subjects who have never talked and/or who have failed to develop relatively normal speech as *nonverbal* in the context of research reviewed by Harris (1975). In cases where there is a history of language, the distinction is somewhat blurred. However, the researcher should carefully evaluate the subject's language over a variety of situations to determine if the mutism is select or a more pervasive language disorder (Miller, 1978b).

Another problem encountered in the literature relates to the frequency of speech across various situations or environments. Some researchers have included low frequency of speech in some situations (and normal speech in other situations) as elective mutism (e.g., Calhoun & Koenig, 1973; Straughan, Potter & Hamilton, 1965). Recognizing this issue, Williamson, Sewell, Sanders, Haney, and White (1977b) proposed the term *reluctant speech* to cover these cases. The authors note:

> A related speaking problem which has not received much attention can be described as "reluctant speech". It differs from elective mutism for though there is a normal frequency of speech under one set of stimulus conditions, there is a very low frequency of speech in others. Examples of reluctant speech are a child who seldom

speaks to certain persons, e.g., adults, or a child who will not spontaneously speak to others but will answer questions [p. 151].

Sanok and Ascione (1979) expanded on this perspective and offered a comparison of elective mutism, reluctant speech, and suppressed speech across various environments (see Figure 1.1).

Unfortunately, employing the term *reluctant* also has problems. In addition to the possible inclusion of a variety of behavior patterns (e.g., presumably withdrawn children with a low frequency of spontaneous talking could be included), it appears that the term *reluctant* conveys (as does *elective*) a connotation of subject-mediated behavior control and consequently adds little to a careful behavior analysis of the situation (cf. Piersel & Kratochwill, 1981). Indeed Sanok and Ascione (1979) are critical of the term "elective mutism" because the term implies covert control residing within the child. The same argument can be advanced against the term "reluctant."

Other behavioral writers have included selective mutism as part of a more general anxiety state and avoidance behaviors, discussing it with other child disorders such as school phobia and social withdrawal (cf. Richards & Siegel, 1978). Various professionals have found that providing suitable definitions of anxiety states and withdrawal behaviors is also a difficult task (e.g., Gelfand, 1979; Marks, 1969; McReynolds, 1978; Miller, Barrett, & Hampe, 1974; Quay, 1972; Ross, 1974). Richards and Siegel (1978) found favor with the definitional

| | Environment 1 | Environment 2 | Environment X |
|---|---|---|---|
| **ELECTIVE MUTISM** | No Speech | Normal Frequency | No Speech or Normal Frequency |
| **RELUCTANT SPEECH** | Low Frequency | Normal Frequency | Low Frequency or Normal Frequency |
| **SUPPRESSED SPEECH** | Low Frequency | Low Frequency | Low Frequency |

FIG. 1.1.   A comparison of elective mutism, reluctant speech, and suppressed speech. (Source: Sanok, R. L., & Ascione, F. R. Behavioral interventions for childhood elective mutism: An evaluative review. *Child Behavior Therapy*, 1979, *1*, 49-68. Reproduced by permission).

approach of Miller et al. (1974), wherein a phobia is characterized as a fear that: (1) is out of proportion to the demands of the situation; (2) cannot be explained or reasoned away; (3) is beyond voluntary control; (4) leads to an avoidance of a feared situation; (5) persists over an extended period of time; (6) is unadaptive; and (7) is not age or stage specific (p. 90). In characterizing anxiety states and avoidance behaviors, Richards and Siegel (1978) note:

> There is a good deal of overlap between anxiety states and avoidance behaviors, of course, with the choice of one or the other labels frequently reflecting a matter of emphasis. Anxiety states usually involve avoidance, and avoidance behaviors usually involve anxiety, but negative emotional states are more pronounced in the anxiety disorders. In turn, withdrawal behaviors and social or intellectual skill deficits are more pronounced in the avoidance disorders. This chapter moves among related terms such as fear, anxiety, phobia, and avoidance in a manner that may well horrify purists: nevertheless, beyond mirroring the shifts of emphasis noted above, the promising behavioral treatment procedures for these overlapping behavior disorders are overlapping themselves and therefore warrant this style of presentation and organization [p. 276].

Thus, we see that these authors are prompted to discuss behavioral problems that have been treated with behavioral techniques whatever the specific classification might be. In this regard, various behavioral programs have been useful for treating withdrawn children, particularly in the area of social skill deficits (cf. Gelfand, 1979), and these procedures are very important in the treatment of selective mutism (see Chapter 7). The interested reader is also referred to more detailed reviews and theoretical discussions on avoidance behaviors in children (e.g., Achenbach, 1974; Clarizio & McCoy, 1976; Gelfand, 1979; Quay, 1972; Ross, 1974).

Perhaps the most important issue in assessment and diagnosis is to conduct a careful behavior analysis of the child's verbal behaviors. The mutism could then be defined in the context of zero occurrence or low-frequency occurrence in certain stimulus situations (e.g., Wulbert et al., 1973). Such a definition is focused directly on differential responding under different stimulus conditions and takes into account stimulus control, which refers to the extent to which the probability of a response is controlled by the presence or absence of a stimulus. Those individuals seeking a more formal classification scheme could easily adopt the sociobehavioral approach outlined by McReynolds (1978). In this regard, selective mutism could be "diagnosed" along the dimensions listed in Table 1.3. Thus a child's selective mutism behaviors might be identified by a family member for behavior change where the disturbance is one of deficit in frequency (and duration or magnitude) in the motor action system. The term *selective mutism* appears to cover the vast majority of cases reviewed in this book. Again, it must be stressed that a careful operational definition of the behavior should be provided after a behavioral analysis of many environmental factors (e.g., home, school, parents, teachers, peers, and so forth). Further guidelines on treatment are presented in Chapter 7.

## LANGUAGE AND SPEECH PROBLEMS

A great deal of research has been published on a variety of procedures to establish speech in nonverbal children and adults (see Schiefelbusch 1978a, 1978b, for an overview). In the past, the term *nonverbal* has generally been limited to intellectually retarded clients who are mute or have minimal functional speech (cf. Harris, 1975). Typically, such clients do not have a repertoire of speech responses, and so a variety of procedures are employed to establish functional verbalizations (e.g., Carrier & Peak, 1977; Guess, Sailor, & Baer, 1977). For example, Harris (1975) reviewed operant conditioning techniques that have been successfully used to teach nonverbal children the skills necessary for functional language. A typical sequence of training involves attention, nonverbal imitation, verbal imitation, and functional speech.

The work of O. Ivar Lovaas and his associates at the University of California at Los Angeles with autistic children represents one of the most programmatic attempts to develop and evaluate treatments for these children. In these programs the children receive treatment for many hours each day. Various treatment procedures are used (e.g., reinforcement in the form of food and praise, extinction, negative reinforcement, punishment, and so on) to modify many different behaviors. Many of the specific problems include the development of receptive and productive speech. The treatment procedures are aimed at developing a functional repertoire of verbal responses.

Although there has been a heterogeneous population included under the umbrella term *nonverbal* (e.g., retarded, autistic), children displaying selective mutism are not included within the general rubric *nonverbal*. The reason is that the latter are considered to have a full repertoire of responses, but have difficulty identifying the discriminative stimuli for speech (Harris, 1975). This feature is also used to distinguish between autistic and adult psychiatric patients who are functionally mute (e.g., Isaacs, Thomas, & Goldiamond, 1960; Sherman, 1963, 1969).

Because mutism represents a problem in the lack of speech under certain stimulus conditions, it is useful to distinguish it from some common problems discussed in the speech pathology literature. Selective mutism might also be distinguished from functional aphonias and dysphonias, two disorders that are presumed to result from improper use of the vocal mechanism and that have an alleged psychoneurotic origin (cf. Marshall & Watts, 1975). Functional dysphonia is commonly classified as the inability of the patient to approximate his or her vocal folds in an optimum manner, with the approximation being either too lax or too tight. In addition, the patient frequently complains of such problems as throat "fullness," pain in the laryngeal area, dryness in the mouth while talking, neck tightness, and the like—which are usually related to vocal fatigue. The patient with functional aphonia frequently is described as having no voice at all, but manages a whisper for most social situations (Boone, 1966).

In both cases of these disorders, an individual's voice problem can be disproportionately severe with regard to any recognized degree of laryngeal involvement, or there may be no apparent alteration in structure detected by laryngoscopic examination. Such cases led Aronson, Peterson, and Liten (1964) to postulate that a number of functional voice disorders reflect changes in psychoneurotic or psychotic mental states (see also Aronson, 1969). These also include spastic dysphonia (Critchley, 1939; Heaver, 1959; Kiml, 1963), ventricular dysphonia (Brodnitz, 1959; Freud, 1962; Jackson & Jackson, 1935), and hysterical aphonia (Barton, 1960; Clerf & Braceland, 1942; Wilson, 1962; Winkelman, 1937). Treatment has consisted of physical manipulation and stimulation of the laryngeal mechanism by the laryngologist (Babcock, 1942; Froschels, 1955; Macmahon, 1932), referral by the laryngologist to the psychiatrist (Barlow, 1930; Barton, 1960), or referral by the laryngologist or psychiatrist to the speech pathoiogist (Ellis, 1959; Willmore, 1959). Some speech pathologists have reported the benefits of voice therapy in conjunction with behavior therapy techniques with functional aphonia cases (Bangs & Freidinger, 1950; Boone, 1966; Gray, England, & Mahoney, 1965; Marshall & Watts, 1975; Walton & Black, 1959).

It is possible that there has been some relation between selective mutism and functional aphonia, although this has never been clearly articulated in the clinical literature. Although selective mutism does not typically involve a physical disability such as vocal nodules, contact ulcers, or polyps, its behavior characteristics may be similar to some forms of functional aphonia postulated to be due to "emotional disturbance." It is also possible that the mutism may be specific to certain situations, whereas functional aphonia is more pervasive in the client's functioning. When the latter is not the case, the distinction is blurred. By whatever name, and with the knowledge that behavior therapy procedures could be used in treating functional aphonia (cf. Boone, 1966; Jackson & Wallace, 1974), the treatment strategy is perhaps the most useful dimension on which to focus. For example, reinforcement and punishment contingencies have been shown to be effective in modifying voice loudness (e.g., Bangs & Freidinger, 1950; Jackson & Wallace, 1974; Walton & Black, 1959), and such procedures have also been applied to treatment of selective mutism.

## SUMMARY AND CONCLUSIONS

This chapter has presented an overview of some issues in diagnosis and classification of selective mutism. Traditional diagnostic systems such as the DSMS, WHO, ICD, AND GAP have not been very helpful in providing a useful classification scheme. The affiliation with the intrapsychic disease model, in addition to the reliability and validity problems of these schemes, renders them problematic. Particularly when these schemes are applied to the problem of selective mutism, they do not yield information useful for treatment.

Alternative systems based on a more overt behavioral approach to classification seem promising in future work on childhood behavioral disorders. In addition to a potentially greater empirical foundation for these approaches, they more closely link diagnosis to assessment and treatment efforts. In providing a classification category for selective mutism, it appears useful to focus on overt behavioral manifestations such as frequency of speech in various situations, patterns of social withdrawal, social skill deficits, and so forth. Generally such a scheme could fit into a sociobehavioral conceptualization in which behavioral excesses and deficits are assessed. Such a system is compatible to most forms of assessment and classification already used in behavior therapy. Nevertheless, empirical work elucidating the parameters of this and other behavioral approaches is clearly indicated.

# 2 Intrapsychic Approaches to the Study of Abnormal Behavior

The global field of behavior and personality assessment and treatment has a long and stormy history. It is a careful understanding of this history that provides a more general perspective on the evolution of certain practices and on why certain techniques were accepted or rejected in practice. Central to this understanding is consideration about the myriad of notions about the nature of humankind and explanations for human behavior (Rhodes & Paul, 1978). Personality theory provides diverse conceptions, depending on the theory one embraces (cf. Hall & Lindzey, 1970; Mischel, 1976; Pervin, 1975), but for our purposes the various approaches can be grouped according to whether behavior is viewed primarily as a product of attributes, states, or traits that lie within the individual or whether behavior is largely influenced by environmental factors. Although there are clearly gray areas in between these two somewhat different perspectives on human functioning, they provide an important contrast for organization of research and treatment of selective mutism.

The research and treatment literature on selective mutism generally falls into an intrapsychic or behavioral approach. An understanding of selective mutism within the intrapsychic perspective requires a review of some major tenets of this orientation to personality theory and assessment. This is the primary objective of Chapter 2.

## INTRAPSYCHIC PERSPECTIVES

One traditional perspective on personality theory is that the individual's behavior is a function of forces acting from within the person. Such forces can include drives, needs, motives, impulses, traits, and so forth. In this paradigm, deviant or abnormal behavior is said to result from a dysfunction or disease process in personality or the development of maladaptive traits.

This view of personality is generally referred to as an *intrapsychic* approach because forces within the individual are said to cause or determine certain behavior. Actually, two major versions of the intrapsychic approach have been dominant in explaining behavior, both normal and abnormal (Kazdin, 1975, 1978a). These two approaches include the *medical* or *disease model* and *trait theory*.

## Medical Model

One form of the intrapsychic approach has commonly been referred to as a medical or disease model because it bears similarity to dominant practices of the medical profession in treating physical diseases (see discussion in Chapter 1). The medical model has been applied in either a literal or metaphorical sense (cf. Phillips et al., 1975). Whereas those subscribing to the literal view assume that symptom classification associated with specific disorders will lead to the discovery of their biological sources and cures, those who hold a metaphorical view do not accept the postulate of a biological causation for psychological disorders. In contrast, they view the overt features of deviant behavior as expressions of deeply ingrained patterns of habits or states. Thus, the medical model—both in its *physiological* features, such as chemical intervention (e.g., prescribing medication for mutism, hyperactivity, schizophrenia) and in its *interpersonal* aspects, such as the psychoanalytic approach—perceives the problem behavior as a deviation from natural occurrence within the person.

In medical practice, certain conditions within the person (e.g., disease, brain dysfunction) account for various symptoms (e.g., perceptual disorders) observed in behavior. In this context, treatment of the symptom is insufficient, because the underlying disease process is causing the problem and so must be treated directly. Within the medical model orientation to understanding human functioning, behavior is considered to reflect underlying components that form personality. Deviant behavior is likewise said to be caused by some underlying defect in basic personality. By extending the analogy from medicine to psychology, it is argued that treatment of the behavior (i.e., symptom) may not cure the real problem.

Freud's (1856–1939) psychoanalytic theory of personality provides one example of the medical model in psychological/psychiatric practice. Although it is commonly believed that psychoanalytic theory is dead, Silverman (1976) suggested that reports of its death have been greatly exaggerated. In addition to the research reviewed by Silverman (1976), Chapter 3 of this volume presents a number of recent studies suggesting that it is a major orientation in the treatment of childhood mutism. Moreover, as noted in Chapter 1, the medical model is a major guiding conceptualization of DSM-III and the clinical practice of psychiatry. In addition to its major influence on contemporary conceptualizations and treatment of abnormal behavior, behavior modification (see Chapter 4) can be viewed as a reaction to many of its basic tenets, and specifically to the notion that intrapsychic conflicts cause deviant behavior (Kazdin, 1978a).

Psychoanalytic theory generally adheres to the medical model by emphasizing that underlying psychological drives cause various behaviors. Behavior is said to be traced to manifestations of unconscious personality processes. The unconscious aspect of psychoanalytic theory pervades the model. Pervin (1975) notes:

> the psychoanalytic concept of the unconscious suggests that a significant portion of our behavior, perhaps the major one, is determined by unconscious forces, and that much of our energy is devoted either to finding acceptable expressions of unconscious ideas or to keeping them unconscious. The concept of the unconscious is deeply embedded in the rest of psychoanalytic theory. Although many new concepts were added as the theory developed, the concept of the unconscious has always remained as part of the framework for the entire theory [p. 157].

In addition to the commonly used term *medical model,* the Freudian view is frequently referred to as the *psychodynamic* view. Dynamics refer to certain phenomena that are explained by referring to energy forces and their relation to motion, growth, and change in physical matter. In Freudian dynamic psychology, behavior is described in terms of psychological energies or basic forces, drives, and impulses and their interrelation. These notions are directly reflected in Freud's (1933) writings, as this example shows:

> One might compare the relation of the ego to the id with that between a rider and his horse. The horse provides the locomotive energy, and the rider has the prerogative of determining the goal and of guiding the movements of his powerful mount toward it. But all too often in the relations between the ego and the id we find a picture of the less ideal situation in which the rider is obliged to guide his horse in the direction in which it itself wants to go [p. 108].

Psychoanalytic theory traces the child's development to psychological impulses that are expressed at various stages. Freud's theory is essentially biologically oriented and is concerned with the derivation of pleasure from specific body zones at different ages (Endler, Boulter, & Osser, 1976). The basic stages are the oral, anal, phallic, latency, and genital. Abnormal development represents a fixation of problems at a particular stage. Diverse behaviors can be traced to the expression of a few psychological forces to which they owe their origin. An interpretation from the psychodynamic literature in explaining "selective mutism" provides an example of this perspective. After examining cases of "elective" mutism, Salfield, Lond, and Dusseldorf (1950) concluded that mutism "can be understood as a fixation at an early infantile level on which an apprehended danger situation is met by refusal to speak [p. 1031]." A further example is the conceptualization of selective mutism by Elson, Pearson, Jones, and Schumacher (1965):

> The symptom complex or syndrome of elective mutism is a neurotic symptom compromise between the indirect expression of the aggressive id wish to destroy the ambivalent mother or mother substitute, and between the archaic superego punishment against this unacceptable and intolerable id wish. Thus, there results a displacement of hostility to less threatening figures such as teachers and other adults [p. 186].

It should be noted that psychoanalytic theory basically focuses on the explanation of an individual's thoughts and feelings at any moment. Overt behavior is thus a primary representation of what one is thinking. Psychoanalytic psychologists emphasize the importance of knowing a person's thoughts; focusing on behavior is perceived as inadequate in assessment. Generally, the basic concepts of psychoanalytic theory are formulated as follows (Baldwin, 1967):

> 1. Instinctual drives energize all human functioning.
> 2. The problem is to show how these instinctual drives energize the particular behavior that maximizes gratification.
> 3. Two major influences set limits on gratification of drives: Reality, and the social rules as mediated by the superego.
> 4. The ego describes the machinery that achieves, more or less effectively, this maximal gratification. It gradually develops structures that channel the discharge of cathexis through cognitive activity, repression, and other defense mechanisms [p. 323].

## Criticisms of the Psychoanalytic Approach

Over the years a variety of criticisms have been levied against psychoanalytic theory (cf. Baldwin, 1967; Kazdin, 1978a; Mikulas, 1978; Mischel, 1976; Pervin, 1975; Stuart, 1970). A basic criticism of psychoanalytic theory is that it focuses upon thoughts and feelings as the real data, and these may be relatively inaccessible. Although one may not discard the theory based on this assumption alone, it poses real methodological problems. Frequently the definitions of its terms that are necessary for scientific validation have not been operationalized (see Chapter 6 for specific examples). As Baldwin (1967) noted, "To a large degree, this failure in operational definitions depends on the fact that the focus of the theory is on thoughts and feelings rather than on overt behavior [p. 384]." Although some of the constructs are relatively well defined, they remain too removed from observable and measurable behavior to be of great empirical use (Pervin, 1975). Sears and his associates (Sears, Rau, & Alpert, 1965) stated the problem nicely:

> We became acutely aware of the differences between the purely descriptive statement of a psychodynamic process and a testable theory of behavioral development.

Psychoanalytic theory contained suggestions for the latter, but it did not specify the conditions under which greater or lesser degrees of any particular behavioral product of identification would occur [p. 241].

Actually, a major problem appears to be a failure to establish operational definitions of terms (and the failure to make explicit the relations and the quantitative estimates among phenomena), rather than the focus on thoughts and feelings. Indeed, it has been the more careful operational definition of various internal events (covert behaviors) that has allowed study of these phenomena within the cognitive behavior modification approach (cf. Bandura, 1976; Thoresen & Mahoney, 1974).

A second problem with the psychoanalytic model, and particularly Freud's energy model, is that it makes many things equivalent. Also, there is a reductionistic quality to the theory that tends to suggest that virtually everything is an expression of sexual and aggressive instincts (Pervin, 1975). As Pervin (1975) has noted, the Freudian view that the infant's sucking at the breast of the mother is the model for every love relation fails to give adequate attention to differences between various love relationships (e.g., child vs. adult, love of mate vs. love of friend, and so forth).

A third criticism of psychoanalytic theory is that it has been difficult to criticize due to its proponents' insistence that it can only be validated through the actual process of psychoanalysis. To put the control of criticism in the hands of individuals with vested interests in the particular model is less than objective science. Moreover, the tendency of proponents of the theory to answer criticisms by attributing them to psychodynamic concepts (e.g., resistance, repression) is generally unacceptable from a scientific perspective.

Another problem is that the theory is often difficult to test, aside from the aforementioned problems with the lack of operational definitions. Generally, the theory fails to state which behaviors will occur given certain sets of circumstances. Thus, in the absence of such statements, the theory does not leave itself open to empirical test (Pervin, 1975).

Finally, there has been a lack of convincing research support for its central assumptions. Part of the problem has been the absence of a rigorous single-case research methodology in psychoanalytic theory. Many applied research strategies within this model have involved case studies that have many methodological flaws (cf. Hersen & Barlow, 1976; Kratochwill, 1978). Of course, research in psychoanalytic theory is not limited to a single-case approach. Multiunit designs have been used in theoretical and applied psychoanalytic research endeavors.

Despite some headway in the research area (e.g., Silverman, 1976), there remain many problems with the model, including the difficulty in verifying many of its propositions scientifically, inconsistencies within the theory itself and in the therapeutic procedures derived from the theory, and lack of empirical support in areas where research has been conducted (cf. Stuart, 1970). Although there have been revisions and additions in Freudian theory that give a greater role to environmental determinants (Hall & Lindzey, 1970), the approach remains remarkably the same and not radically altered by followers who have supplanted Freud's views.[1]

## Trait Theory

Like the Freudian view, the trait theory orientation provides a further example of the intrapsychic position. In trait theory, personality structures are said to account for behavior (Mischel, 1968, 1974). Although many trait approaches developed years ago, the orientation also represents a major force in current-day practice. In a recent interview, Cattell indicated (Krug, 1978):

> The modern approach [to personality testing] says let's find out what personality structure we should be measuring first and then find devices to measure them. . . . In my own work we started with a list of all the personality traits that existed in the English language. We had available new, powerful techniques like factor analysis for analyzing the interrelationships among these traits empirically and finding the factors of major importance which explained the relationships among the literally thousands of traits people use to describe personality. It has taken us 30 or 40 years to bring the personality area to the same precision as people like Spearman and Thurstone did in the ability area, but we now have a number of modern questionnaires which measure well replicated personality dimensions [p. 29].

Traits generally refer to consistent and relatively enduring ways of behaving that are used to distinguish one individual from another. Traits are inferred from behaviors (usually measured on tests) and are said to persist and be consistent over time and across various situations. Some personality researchers have taken the position that people can most typically be characterized in terms of 8 to 10 well-chosen traits or constructs (cf. Allport, 1937; Kelly, 1955). Although this assumption may appear simplistic, some writers suggest that this approach has proven productive as a means of advancing our understanding of social behavior and, thus, has a measure of justification (cf. Hogan, DeSota, & Solano, 1977). Although different trait theorists disagree on what traits explain certain be-

---

[1]Whereas the psychoanalytic theory of development gives major attention to the first 5 years of life and to the development of instincts, ego psychologists (e.g., Erikson, 1963) have given greater attention to other developments during the early years and to significant developments that take place during the latency and genital stages (cf. Pervin, 1975). Moreover, in more recent developments (e.g., Erikson, 1963) of psychoanalytic theory, the role of rational processes in the individual's development is emphasized, and more attention is being paid to psychosocial development than in previous years (Endler et al., 1976). Nevertheless, the major revisions have been conceptualized within the basic Freudian model.

haviors, they all generally adhere to the position that there are behavioral patterns that are consistent and that these patterns are expressions or signs of underlying traits.

## Criticisms of Trait Theory

Traits have always had a major role in communication among people wherein they serve as summary labels to represent consistent patterns of behavior. This is reflected in the foregoing quote from Cattell wherein he employed various labels to initiate research on traits. For example, one may label an individual as "kind." Such an individual may be observed to display "kindness" in certain situations (e.g., the individual is observed helping an elderly citizen across the street) and is labeled as a kind person. Presumably, this "kindness" could be a trait that finds expression in diverse situations and remains consistent across time. Used in this context, traits have served a useful function in a language system. It is when they are used to *explain* behavior that they cause some problems. Kazdin (1975, pp. 4–5) listed three reasons why traits are inadequate as explanations for behavior.

First, it is presumed that traits can be inferred from overt behavior(s). A person who behaves in a hostile fashion may be considered to have the trait "hostility." The problem that occurs is that the trait that has been inferred from behavior is used to explain the behavior; that is, the reason the person is hostile is postulated to be the trait "hostility." This account of traits is essentially circular. A meaningful criterion for traits would have to be determined independently of the behaviors they are supposed to explain. Critics of this argument raise the point that traits are not inferred from a single behavior performed in one situation, but from different behaviors in a variety of situations. Rather, traits are inferred from a large number of individuals with various traits or various amounts of a certain trait consistent over time and situations.

A counterargument can be advanced within the context of the criticism. There is some evidence to suggest that individuals do not always perform consistently across a variety of situations and over time, as would be predicted from the trait position (Mischel, 1968). Moreover, different behaviors that are considered to make up a general trait often are not highly correlated. In our hostility example, various behaviors that make up such a personality trait may not be performed consistently. The person may act in a hostile fashion in one situation with a certain person, but may not act in this manner in other situations. Thus, a person's response may change as the situations change. There is some evidence to suggest that children display different patterns of aggressive behavior (Bandura & Walters, 1963) and social behavior (Redd, 1969) depending on the person with whom they are interacting. Moreover, it may be that the consistency that a person *perceives* in someone's behavior appears to come from conceptions of the perceiver rather from the person he or she is observing (e.g., Dornbusch, Hastorf, Richardson, Muzzy, & Vreeland, 1965).

Another criticism of a trait explanation of behavior is that the antecedent conditions that explain traits are often not explained. A behavior is not really explained by relating it to an underlying trait until the trait has been accounted for (Skinner, 1953). Such underlying concepts, which are used to explain behavior in this fashion, are called "explanatory fictions" or "mental way stations" by Skinner. Although attributing behavior to a trait or state appears to provide an explanation of behavior, the traits or states are not expanded; so no actual scientific explanation has been provided.

A final criticism of the trait position relates to the system used to assess traits. Traits are usually measured with some type of standardized assessment instrument such as an IQ test or projective device. The score one obtains on a test is usually thought to reflect the property of the individual assumed to be measured by the test (e.g., intelligence from an intelligence test). This sets up a test–trait fallacy (Tryon, 1979) that begins with the faulty assumption that: (1) test scores are trait measures; (2) trait measures are basic properties of the person; and (3) test scores reflect basic properties of the person. Tryon (1979) notes: "This sequence essentially converts a dependent variable into an independent variable; hence a measurement is reified into a causal force. It should also be emphasized that the unsound logic of drawing inferences about *ability* on the basis of observed performance is integral to the test–trait fallacy [p. 402]."

Despite the criticism of the intrapsychic approach, it is clear that the theory and various forms of assessment are clearly alive and "well." In fact, even if it can be agreed that individuals are not adhering to an intrapsychic theoretical position, the use of various assessment devices within this general paradigm is quite pervasive. The influence is most keenly felt in the areas of assessment and diagnosis. In Chapter 1, the use of conventional diagnostic categories was reviewed. This sytems represents one major influence of the psychodynamic orientation in clinical practice. We now turn our attention to the assessment of personality within the intrapsychic orientation.

## ASSESSMENT WITHIN THE INTRAPSYCHIC ORIENTATION

The intrapsychic orientation toward human behavior has strongly influenced the assessment practices of psychologists, psychiatrists, social workers, and others involved in providing treatment services for various personality disorders. Because individuals are assumed to have underlying states or traits that account for behavior, emphasis has been placed on determining underlying personality rather than on observing behavior directly. The search for underlying ability measure is perhaps most apparent in the use of intelligence tests for screening school-age children for special classes. Alfred Binet's (1857–1911) work in the area of achievement testing provided a major impetus to the development of psychological tests for personality. Nevertheless, much of Binet's work has been misrepresented as being solely a testing role (see Sarason, 1976).

Psychoanalytic theory played a major role in shaping the focus of personality assessment. Psychoanalysis stimulated the formulation of theories of personality that generated unique methods of personality assessment and helped to unify independently devised methods of personality assessment that developed without allegiance to certain theoretical positions (Kazdin, 1978a).

Clearly, there are now a variety of personality theories that differ from the psychoanalytic model, but despite great diversity, they can be labeled as "non-behavioral," and they share certain common characteristics. These characteristics generally include a conception of personality as consisting of relatively stable and interrelated motives, characteristics, and dynamics that underlie and determine overt behaviors. In this conception, assessment must focus on understanding underlying dynamics.

Within this orientation, a variety of procedures have been developed. Indeed, personality research in the United States has traditionally relied on personality assessment for its data base. Such measurement devices as the F scale (Adorno, Frenkel-Brunswik, Levinson, & Sanford, 1950); the Minnesota Multiphasic Personality Inventory (MMPI; Hathaway & McKinley, 1943); the TAT-based (Thematic Apperception Test) measures of need (Achievement) (McClelland, Atkinson, Clark, & Lowell, 1953); and the California Psychological Inventory (CPI; Gough, 1969) have represented subdisciplines within the study of personality psychology. These forms of assessment devices can generally be catagorized as indirect measurement strategies (cf. Hersen & Barlow, 1976; Mischel, 1972). Traditional assessment relies on a "sign" approach, as opposed to the "sample" orientation taken by behavioral researchers and clinicians (Goldfried, 1976; Goldfried & Kent, 1972). Within the traditional framework, the nature of the situation in which the individual is functioning is of less interest in the assessment than are underlying motives, dynamics, or structural components. Goldfried (1976) noted:

> The basic difference between traditional and behavioral assessment procedures is best reflected in a distinction originally made by Goodenough in 1949, when she drew the comparison between a "sign" and "sample" approach to the interpretation of tests. When test responses are viewed as a sample, one assumes that they parallel the way in which a person is likely to behave in a nontest situation. Thus, if a person responds aggressively on a test, one assumes that the aggression also

occurs in other situations as well. When test responses are viewed as signs, an inference is made that the performance is an indirect or symbolic manifestation of some other characteristic [p. 283].

Goldfried and Kent (1972) have compared traditional and behavioral assessment with specific focus on the assumptions associated with each. A major difference relates to the levels of inference associated with the two approaches. Generally, the traditional approach has a greater degree of inferential activity in the assessment process. For example, in using a traditional test of personality, a *method assumption* relates to the belief that the test scores (e.g., TAT responses) are only minimally affected by artifacts associated with the measurement and scoring process itself. At the next level of inference, one must assume that the testing procedure has accurately sampled from the population of potential responses that presumably indicate the personality characteristics associated with some problem. At the final level of inference, an interpretation is commonly made regarding the nature of the personality characteristics or construct manifested by the test responses themselves (see Goldfried, 1976; Goldfried & Kent, 1972; for further discussion of these issues).

A final feature of traditional assessment that is relevant to consider is its relation to a treatment program (e.g., Bandura, 1969; Ciminero, 1977; Goldfried & Pomeranz, 1968; Kanfer & Phillips, 1970; Peterson, 1968; Stuart, 1970). As was noted in Chapter 1, formal diagnosis is typically made subsequent to some type of assessment in the traditional or psychodynamic model. Although there may be some relation between this assessment and diagnosis, there appears to be little relation between traditional assessment and treatment. Traditional assessment usually occurs prior to (and sometimes after) treatment, but has only an indirect role in a particular treatment strategy.

## Limitations of Traditional Assessment

Some of the aforementioned features of traditional intrapsychic assessment could be construed as limitations when compared to behavioral assessment. For example, a low correspondence between assessment and treatment seems to be a major limitation on logical grounds alone. There has been increasing pessimism regarding the utility and importance of many intrapsychic measurement systems. Hogan et al. (1977) identified five sources of problems that are leading to skepticism regarding personality tests in general (pp. 255-256).

1. The concept of a trait as a unit of analysis in personality research has been criticized in recent years (cf. Fiske, 1974; Jones, Kanouse, Kelley, Nisbett, Valins, & Weiner, 1971; Mischel, 1968; Peterson, 1968). The assumption that certain tests measure traits has led to less faith in their relevance for research and practice (see also Tryon, 1979).

2. Some critics have noted that personality tests don't work very well, that validity coefficients approach .30 as an upper-limit bound, and that social behavior is primarily a function of situational contingencies (e.g., Mischel, 1968).

3. A review of various English-language journals of personality and social psychology reveals that experimentation has become the predominant methodology. Most experimental paradigms have revealed group differences and have minimized the effects of individual differences. This emphasis has led to a general decline in test-based personality research.

4. Personality measurement through indirect measurement strategies originally was developed to aid psychiatric diagnosis. Some approaches (e.g., behavior therapy) do not depend exclusively on this form of assessment. Even nonbehaviorally oriented clinicians have increasingly noted that insanity is in the eyes of the beholder, that mental illness is best understood in terms of labeling theory, and that neurotic and psychotic syndromes discoverable through assessment methods say more about the therapist's belief systems than about the client's behavior (cf. Goffman, 1961; Kelly, 1955; Rosenhan, 1973; Scheff, 1973; Szasz, 1974).

5. Tests tend to encourage "mindless" research in that marginally competent investigators can appear productive by administering a number of tests to a population and then discovering significant relations among the resulting correlations without holding any substantive a priori hypotheses.

Hogan et al. (1977) take the position that most of the assumptions or claims of test critics don't apply to personality *research* as it is currently practiced. They argue that personality assessment is a logical extension of personality theory and that its role is nonoverlapping but complementary to that of experimental social psychology in the study of behavior. Thus, research on personality assessment and experimental research should be encouraged.

It is difficult to argue with the call for more research. Despite these issues, the debate continues. Whereas proponents of traditional assessment argue that evaluative studies of traits and diagnostic measures are inadequate or inappropriate (cf. Alker, 1972; Holt, 1970; Wachtel, 1973a, 1973b), projective test proponents argue that current research strategies are far too primitive to examine certain personality dynamics or nonpsychometric aspects of projective techniques (cf. Holzberg, 1960; McCully, 1965; Sarason, 1976). Critics of traditional assessment cite negative results concerning reliability, validity, and utility and question the continued usage of such techniques (e.g., Bem, 1972; Bersoff, 1973; Chapman & Chapman, 1971; Jensen, 1969; Mischel, 1968, 1973a, 1973b). Moreover, as has already been noted, the presumption that test scores provide measures of enduring and generalized characteristics of an individual labeled "traits" represent a test–trait fallacy (Tryon, 1979). Nevertheless, one issue that should be raised in this regard is to what degree all these issues influence training and practice.

## PERVASIVENESS OF TRADITIONAL TESTING
## PRACTICES

Klopfer and Taulbee (1976) began their review of ''projective tests'' by asking if theirs would be the last time that a chapter on projective tests would appear in the *Annual Review of Psychology.* Likely, their question will be answered with a negative response. These authors note that there were more than 500 journal articles pertaining to projective techniques during the review period 1971 through 1974, not including a number of books published or revised. Moreover, in comparison of three national surveys (Louttit & Browne, 1947; Lubin, Wallis, & Paine, 1971; Sundberg, 1961) of psychological test practices from 1947 to 1971, only minor changes in top-ranking tests are demonstrated. For example, during the decade between the last two surveys, the Rorschach dropped in rank from first to second place, replaced by the Wechsler Adult Intelligence Scale (WAIS) in the top spot; the TAT moved from fourth place to tie with the Bender–Gestalt test for third. Klopfer and Taulbee (1976) conclude their review by indicating:

> The most distinct contribution that projective tests continue to make, however, probably is in revealing aspects of motivation and personality that do not fit neatly into either the self-concept or behavioral category. Creative capacities, hidden resources, potentialities that currently are not in use are variables that sometimes emerge better in projective test performance than through other sources of information. Until clinical psychologists give up an interest in the inner person and abandon their search for probing the depths of the psyche, they probably will continue to use, improve, and rely upon the data derived from projective techniques [p. 563].

More recent information on testing practice continues to support the notion that traditional tests are commonly used. Although Shemberg and Keeley (1970), Thelen and Ewing (1970), and Thelen, Varble, and Johnson (1968) have reported a general decline in testing training (especially among newer psychology training programs) and a shift from projective testing toward objective testing, recent surveys suggest that testing continues to play a substantial role in applied settings (e.g., Levy & Fox, 1975: Wade & Baker, 1977; Wade, Baker, & Hartmann, 1979).

Wade and Baker (1977) surveyed 500 clinical psychologists about their use and opinions of psychological tests. The results showed that both objective and projective tests are used by clinical psychologists of all major therapeutic orientations with substantial percentages of clients. Clinicians indicated that personal clinical experience with a test was more important in their test-use decisions than pragmatic or psychometric considerations. Moreover, clinicians repeatedly emphasized the subjective, insightful, and experiential nature of the testing process.

Interestingly, the psychometric limitations of tests were recognized, but tests were considered more valuable than suggested by reliability and validity studies, which were typically considered *flawed* or *inaccurate*. Wade and Baker (1977) noted that clinicians are probably unaffected by negative testing research because: (1) there are strong needs to assess (i.e., probably, assessment is reinforced); (2) clinicians accord personal clinical experience greater weight than experimental evidence; and (3) there are a few practical alternatives to tests.

Presumably, a large number of behavior therapists were included in their sample. Indeed, recent surveys indicate that behavior therapy is the second most frequent orientation among clinical psychologists (cf. Garfield & Kurtz, 1976; Wade & Baker, 1977; Wade, Baker, Morton, & Baker, 1978). Moreover, research and treatment innovations in the area of behavior therapy have steadily increased as have the teaching of behaviorally oriented courses in academic institutions (Benassi & Lanson, 1972) and the availability of internship training opportunities (Johnson & Bolstad, 1973). Finally, membership in behavior therapy professional societies (e.g., *Association for Advancement* of Behavior Therapy [AABT] and Behavior Therapy Research Soceity [BTRS]) has increased, as have the number of journals devoted to behaviorally oriented research and therapy journals. In this regard, it would be informative to examine the views and practices of behavior therapists with regard to assessment and treatment.

Wade, Baker, and Hartmann (1979) did just that. They sampled behavior therapists from the AABT (450 responses). The survey revealed that colleges and universities were the predominant work settings of behavior therapists and that the greatest portion of their professional time was allocated to therapy. Treatment was most frequently provided for anxiety, child management problems, marital difficulties, and depression. The most commonly used treatment procedures were operant conditioning, systematic desensitization, and modeling. Although some behavioral assessment strategies were reported (e.g., behavior interviews and observation), traditional interviews and objective and projective personality tests were also frequently used. Behavioral assessment was considered valuable for defining problems and treatment planning, but was often considered impractical in applied settings. The most frequently reported reasons for using personality tests were agency requirements and patient categorization or classification. The interesting implication raised by Wade et al. (1979) is that the most influential factor contributing to the use of nonbehavioral assessment approaches is the *difficulty* of using behavioral strategies in applied settings, a liability cited by almost half the respondents. The implications of the findings were that behavior therapists view behavioral assessment as more relevant to clients' problems than tests, but that practical problems limit the use of behavioral assessment. They suggest that future goal of behavior therapy research would be to develop human engineering systems that permit behavioral assessment to be done more quickly and economically.

## CONCLUDING COMMENTS AND PERSPECTIVES

In this chapter the conceptualization of abnormal behavior within the intrapsychic-disease approach was reviewed across the medical and trait models. Limitations of each of these intrapsychic perspectives were discussed in the context of a contrast to a behavioral approach to treatment. Finally, the intra-psychic assessment paradigm was reviewed and limitations presented.

The traditional intrapsychic-disease model has generally not provided the kind of empirical research base that has been deemed important in the mainstream of psychology. For example, many of the procedures developed from psychoanalytic theory were not based on objective observations and were virtually impossible to replicate because of poorly defined concepts. Support for theoretical claims was based on subjective interpretation, so the method and the results were not part of general scientific method.

Despite the numerous limitations raised in the discussion of the intrapsychic model in dealing with deviant behavior, some positive features can be noted. First, it was apparent that ancient conceptions of deviant behavior attributed behavior problems to supernatural forces or powers. For example, during the colonial period, treatment of deviant behavior was less than human, as this account (Deutsch, 1946) demonstrates:

> The mentally ill were hanged, imprisoned, tortured, and otherwise persecuted as agents of Satan. Regarded as sub-human beings, they were chained in specially devised kennels and cages like wild beasts.... they were incarcerated in work-house dungeons or made to slave as able-bodied paupers, unclassified from the rest. They were left to wander about stark naked, driven from place to place like mad dogs, subjected to whipping as vagrants and rouges [p. 53].

It is also possible that children speaking only to select individuals or in certain situations were said to be possessed by evil spirits. Exorcism may have been the treatment of choice. Thus, a recasting of the deviant individual as mentally ill or diseased likely has yielded more humane treatment of such individuals (Kazdin, 1975). This is usually apparent in the treatment of childhood mutism.

# 3 An Overview of Psychodynamic Research

This chapter presents an overview of the reported research on selective mutism wherein the approach to description and/or treatment involved an intrapsychic or psychodynamic orientation. As noted in Chapter 2, this view holds that personality is an assortment of psychic forces inside the child, including drives, impulses, needs, motives, and personality traits. Thus, the mute behavior will typically be regarded as a dysfunction or "disease" process in personality or the development of maladaptive traits.

## PSYCHODYNAMIC CASE STUDIES

All research and treatment programs for the selective mute child established from the psychodynamic orientation have been descriptive and/or treatment case studies.[1] In the former, writers typically described various characteristics of the child referred for mute behavior, whereas the latter typically included some combination of descriptive information and intervention procedures.

### Historical Characteristics

The psychodynamic literature on selective mutism includes writings from many countries. Prominent among them is Germany, where the earliest and most extensive clinical reports have appeared (Amman, 1958; Arnold & Luchsinger,

---

[1] The research and treatment literature on elective mutism includes a rather large base in foreign journals, with a large frequency in the German literature. Although some of this literature is cited, many of the reports were either unavailable for translation or were not translated. Many of the reports in foreign journals, and in German ones in particular, are written from an intrapsychic orientation, but this is not reflected in the review.

1949; Ehrsam & Hesse, 1956; Furster, 1956; Geiger-Martz, 1951; Gutzmann, 1893; Heinze, 1932; Heuger & Morgenstern, 1927; Kistler, 1927; Kummer, 1953; Kussmaul, 1885; Liebmann, 1898; Lesch, 1934; Mitscherlich, 1952; Nadoleczng, 1926; Pangalila-Ratulangie, 1959; Rothe, 1928; Schepank, 1960; Spieler, 1941, 1944; Stern, 1910; Tramer, 1934, 1949; Tramer & Geiger-Martz, 1952; Treidel, 1894; Treuper, 1897; Wallis, 1957; Waternik & Veder, 1936). The term *elective mutism* is commonly attributed to Tramer (1934), but a number of German writers published papers that descriptively reported cases of ''voluntary'' mute behavior in children (cf. Gutzmann, 1893; Liebmann, 1898; Stern, 1910; Treuper, 1897) and described therapeutic interventions (e.g., hypnosis, suggestion, persuasion) for the mute child (cf. Froschels, 1926; Heuger & Morgenstern, 1927; Kistler, 1927; Lesch, 1934). In an historical survey of the German literature, Von Misch (1952) reported that in 1877, Kussmaul used the term *aphasia voluntaria* to describe individuals of normal intellect who forced themselves into mutism for purposes they refused to disclose (see also Froeschels, Dietrich, & Wilhelm, 1932, for a similar perspective in the American literature). The term *elective mutism* reflects the early psychodynamic orientation through its emphasis on the voluntary or elective component of this behavioral problem. Thus, the child is characterized as choosing or electing to remain mute in certain social situations. This term has generally been retained in the American literature and also transcends therapeutic orientations in that psychodynamic and behavioral researchers have used it to refer to the same pattern of behavior (cf. Kratochwill et al., 1979).

## Descriptive Treatment Reports

Some writers reviewed a large number of school (Parker, Olsen, & Throckmorton, 1960), hospital (e.g., Koch, 1976; Koch & Goodlund, 1973), and clinic (Arajarvi, 1965; Silverman & Powers, 1970; Wright, 1968) cases, providing extensive descriptive information in addition to therapeutic programs. Parker et al. (1960) reviewed the case files from the Tacoma Public Schools (Tacoma, Washington) from September 1947 through January 1959 and found 27 children referred for casework services who did talk at home. As more than 3600 children received casework services during this period, the 13 girls and 14 boys comprised only about .7% of the total population seen. There were no significant differences in incidences of this problem from year to year. As expected, the problem prompted early referrals. Of the 27 children, 19 were referred during kindergarten, 6 during the first 3 months of first grade, and the remaining 2 children almost immediately after they entered the school system in grades two and four.

Review of the 18 more severe cases by Parker et al. (1960) suggested that the ''symptom'' was based upon neurotic factors within the family structure. The following dynamic factors were purportedly significant in the elective mutism (Parker et al., 1960):

1. Mouth injury or mouth trauma at the time a child was learning speech or severe or prolonged illness at the time especially in conjunction with separation from the mother.

2. Family patterns of non-speaking either on the part of parents when they themselves were young, or current patterns of non-speaking as a retaliatory expression of hostility on the part of adults within the family.

3. Unsatisfactory nature of the mother–child relationship. This symbiotic relationship had not been resolved and deep feelings of frustration, with resultant anger, were experienced by both mother and child. The mouth remained cathected since normal infancy gratification had not been achieved [p. 67].

Some behavioral characteristics of these children were also reported. Eleven of the 18 children were reported as not participating in any classroom activities at the time of referral. Several of the youngsters apparently refused to remove their coats or hats and would not enter the classroom without being led.

The therapeutic procedures for these children involved work with the teacher, parents, and child. The social worker frequently met with the teacher and parents to plan an intervention strategy that mainly consisted of discussions of the child's dynamics (e.g., work with the child was "directed toward the development of a more stable and differentiated ego [p. 69]").

The authors report that some use of speech in the classroom was reported in all cases prior to termination of treatment except for 1 boy, who moved. Two cases were terminated in less than 3 months, 6 in from 3 to 9 months, 3 in 1½ to 2 years. Only 1 case remained open over 2 years. At the time of the review, 5 cases were active.

Arajarvi (1965) reported a follow-up of 12 children labeled "selective mute" who were treated from 1952 to 1962 at the children's department of the Neurological and Psychiatric Clinic of the University of Helsinki. The 8 girls and 4 boys had learned to speak normally, but they had stopped speaking to strangers, to their fathers, or at school to the teacher at the age of 4 to 8 years. Although all the children spoke to their mothers, starting school had been difficult, and they were described as shy, inhibited, and passive. Eleven were of normal intelligence, and 1 was diagnosed as mentally retarded.

Table 3.1 shows various characteristics of the group of children. The author notes that 9 children started to speak during the treatment (unspecified) after a period of 2 to 4 weeks; 3 children remained silent during the entire period of hospitalization (they did answer questions in writing); and aggressiveness occurred in 9 children. It can be observed that the treatment ranged from 1 to 8 months. Eight children received some form of individual therapy, with 5 improving from this involvement.

TABLE 3.1
Symptoms Associated with Not-Speaking[a]

| No. and Sex | Spoke | | Stopped Speaking at | Age at Admission | Started to Speak at Hospital after | Duration of Treatment | Follow-up Inquiry after | Speaks Normally |
|---|---|---|---|---|---|---|---|---|
| | Words at | Sentences at | | | | | | |
| 1 girl | 12 mos. | 18 mos. | 7 yrs. | 15 yrs. | — | 5 mos. | 2 y./10 y. | −/+ |
| 2 boy | | 18 mos. | 4 yrs. | 9 yrs. | 3 mos. | 6 mos. | 2 y./10 y. | −/+ |
| 3 girl | 12 mos. | 24 mos. | 7 yrs. | 13 yrs. | — | 2 mos. | 1 y./6 y. | −/+ |
| 4 boy | | 20 mos. | 7 yrs. | 9 yrs. | 2 weeks | 5 mos. | 5 yrs. | + |
| 5 girl | 12 mos. | | (5) 8 yrs. | 15 yrs. | 1 mo. | 2½ mos. | 5 yrs. | + |
| 6 girl | 12 mos. | | 8 yrs. | 15 yrs. | 2 weeks | 3½ mos. | 5 yrs. | + |
| 7 boy | 12 mos. | 24 mos. | 4 yrs. | 8/12 yrs. | — | 8/4 mos. | 2 yrs. | − |
| 8 boy | 12 mos. | 18 mos. | 7 yrs. | 10 yrs. | 3 days | 1 mo. | 3 yrs. | + |
| 9 girl | | 17 mos. | 8 yrs. | 10 yrs. | 4 mos. | 6 mos. | 2 yrs. | + |
| 10 girl | | 24 mos. | 7 yrs. | 8 yrs. | 1 mo. | 5½ mos. | 1 y. | + |
| 11 girl | | 18 mos. | 5 yrs. | 8 yrs. | 3 days | 3 mos. | 1 y. | + |
| 12 girl | 12 mos. | | 7 yrs. | 10 yrs. | 1 week | 1½ mos. | 1 y. | + |

[a]From Arajärvi (1965).

The family background of these children demonstrated considerable deviance. It was reported that the fathers were violent alcoholics, feared by both mothers and children, or reticent, distant, and indifferent toward the children. Moreover, the mothers were characterized as emotionally cold, or depressive and tired, or infantile and apprehensive.

Despite the rather negative family situations of these children, following treatment, 11 of the 12 children were able to speak and go to school. However, only 2 were able to return to their former schools. Seven were returned to their own homes; 3 were placed in foster homes; 1 was placed in a children's home and in a school for the mentally retarded. Although the follow-up shows some positive pattern, it is impossible to attribute these changes on outcome and follow-up to the intervention program. The lack of a specific description of the treatment remains a major limitation in this report.

Over a 7-year period from 1958 to 1965, Wright (1968) evaluated 24 clients, ages 5 to 9 years, who were referred to Hawthorne Center (Northville, Michigan) because of their failure to speak at school. The children were treated for periods varying from a few weeks to 2 years, with the majority being treated for 3 to 4 months. All children were treated initially in an outpatient clinic, and 3 of the 24 cases were subsequently admitted to the inpatient service for periods of 3 to 6 months. Individual psychotherapy (unspecified) was the primary treatment, with school personnel becoming involved at certain points in treatment. Occasionally, rewards were offered for speaking.

There was a great deal of diversity in terms of sex, age of onset, age at time of referral, grade level, and intelligence (see Table 3.2). When a combination of

TABLE 3.2
Characteristics of Children Reviewed by Wright (1968),
Who Demonstrated Selective Mutism in School[a]

| Characteristic | Dimension | Numerical Value | Percentage |
|---|---|---|---|
| Sex of client | Male | 7 | 29 |
| | Female | 17 | 71 |
| Age at onset | 5 yrs | 13 | 54 |
| | 4 yrs | 6 | 25 |
| | 3 yrs | 5 | 21 |
| Age at time of referral | 5 yrs | 6 | 25 |
| | 6 yrs | 6 | 25 |
| | 7 yrs | 8 | 34 |
| | 8 yrs | 2 | 16 |
| | 9 yrs | 2 | 16 |
| Grade level at time of referral | Kindergarten | 11 | 46 |
| | 1st grade | 5 | 21 |
| | 2nd grade | 7 | 29 |
| | 3rd grade | 1 | 4 |
| Intelligence | Defective range | 1 | 4 |
| | Borderline range | 5 | 21 |
| | Dull-normal range | 3 | 12.5 |
| | Normal range | 6 | 25 |
| | Bright-normal range | 3 | 12.5 |
| | Superior range | 5 | 21 |
| | Not tested | 1 | 4 |
| Adjustment at time of follow-up | Excellent | | 21 |
| | Good | | 58 |
| | Fair | | 16 |
| | Poor | | 5 |

[a] After Wright (1968).

problems such as low intelligence, organic factors, thought disorders, and so forth were apparent, the prognosis was poorer, even though many of the clients responded well to treatment. Follow-up data (gathered from 6 months to 7 years later on 19 cases) obtained through interviews suggested that 79% had excellent to good adjustment. Wright (1968) indicated that mutism may be caused by a number of etiological factors, with a dominant underlying neurotic problem common in all cases, particularly a neurotic relationship between child and mother, characterized by dependence and ambivalence coupled with an excessive need to control.

In an extensive follow-up investigation of mute children, Kock and Goodlund (1973) examined the files of 17 children who were diagnosed electively mute while hospitalized in the child psychiatry service at the University of Minnesota.[2]

[2] Analysis of these cases is also presented in Koch (1976).

The authors were able to obtain follow-up data on 13 of the original 17. While at the child psychiatry service, most of the clients were seen individually in psychotherapy sessions (unspecified), and parental counseling was offered where indicated and if possible. It was noted that 3 of the children had reward systems established for speaking and a withdrawal of the usual privileges unless they were requested by the child. Whereas a previous approach of ignoring the mutism had failed, this strategy presumably was effective.

The average length of hospital stay was 14 weeks. At discharge, 3 of the children still demonstrated selective mutism with their physician or other hospital staff, but only 1 refused to talk to anyone outside of family members.

At the time of follow-up, all clients were living at home. The youngest, aged 8 years, had a 4-year follow-up. The remainder of the clients ranged in age from 14 to 21 years, and the average follow-up was 9 years. Both the clients and their parents were interviewed privately and conjointly. The MMPI and an intelligence test were administered, and school reports and data from social agencies and mental health facilities were obtained. The subjects were rated on a 5-point scale (see Table 3.3). The major difficulties for these clients were with socialization, family conflicts, social adjustment, and independence, but generally not mutism. Koch and Goodlund (1973) suggested that the mute children as a group were heterogeneous. However, one child, where continued interaction was absent, became more and more mute over the years and subsequently would not even respond to a structured inpatient approach.

TABLE 3.3

Factors Considered in Determining the Degree of Incapacitation
of 13 Mute Children, Including School Adjustment;
Social Relationships with Parents, Peers, and Siblings;
Autonomous Functioning; and Self-Concept[a]

| Rating on 5-Point Scale | Description | Number of Subjects |
|---|---|---|
| 1. Positive mental health | Above average in total life adjustment | 0 |
| 2. Problem behavior not incapacitating | Behavior within normal limits | 4 |
| 3. Problem behavior mildly incapacitating | Some evidence of interference with life adjustment factors | 2 |
| 4. Problem behaviors moderately incapacitating | Significant impairment of function | 7 |
| 5. Problem behavior severely incapacitating | Requires institutionalization and/or primary support and protection of others | 0 |

[a]After Koch and Goodlund (1973, p. 31).

Silverman and Powers (1970) indicated that many children have been referred to the Virginia Treatment Center for Children (in Richmond) with the symptom of mutism (e.g., schizophrenia, hysterical aphonia, brain damage, degenerative brain diseases, and elective mutism). Using their diagnostic criteria (see Chapter 6, p. 137), five cases were treated for elective mutism. In the first case, Eric, a 13-year-old boy, had not spoken to any adults for 7 years and had not spoken to his parents for 5 years. The only communication he had was with his siblings.

In the case of Dan, a 13-year-old boy, the mutism developed after age 2½, when his father left home and the family situation deteriorated. Sara, approximately age 7, had not spoken to people outside the home since age 3 or 4. Becky was a 7-year-old child who had not spoken for a period of at least 2 years. Charles, age 12, had not spoken publicly for the past 3 years. The authors report:

> It would seem that his symptom began one day in the first grade when he was allegedly told to sit down and shut up. Immediately following this, Charles defecated in his pants and was told to stand outside for the rest of the day. After this incident, he refused to talk publicly to any peers or adults. Up until his admission, he had only continued to converse with his siblings and his parents [p. 185].

Some common features of these five cases include disturbed home environments (e.g., disturbed parents) and marked disturbance in the parent–child relationships (e.g., parent leaving home). Specific therapeutic procedures are lacking in their report, but presumably the clients received psychotherapy. The authors suggested that the surface behavior of mutism has to do with oral difficulties, improverishment of object relationships, inability to tolerate separation, and fear of rejection.

## Treatment Reports

The vast majority of psychodynamic case studies have taken place in clinic settings, with only several occurring in schools (e.g., Browne, Wilson, & Laybourne, 1963; Strait, 1958; Werner, 1945). Two early British reports by writers involved in the treatment of selective mutism showed little promise of developing functional speech (Morris, 1953; Salfield, Lond, & Dusseldorf, 1950). Salfield et al. (1950) reported one case and reviewed some others from their own clinical work as well as from the reports of Tramer (1934, 1949). In one case, Salfield et al. (1950) noted:

> We could demonstrate by recording his voice when he was at play, alone with his brother, that he spoke to him, if only in monosyllables. We have also heard him say "thank you" to the P.S.W. [Psychiatric Social Worker]. When offered two pennies as a present, he did say "thank you" whilst he refused to say so for one penny. Reports that he spoke fluently in the village were also verified [p. 6022].

Although specific descriptions of the treatment procedures are lacking in their report, it was noted that one child was in play therapy for over a year. The child eventually talked freely at home and to strangers, but he continued to remain mute at school. Several observations were provided after reviewing their own and other cases: (1) Elective mutism occurs between 3 and 5 years of age; (2) no mental defect appears present; (3) a frequent familial factor occurs; (4) great resistance to treatment is common; and (5) there may be an early psychological or compound trauma. Mutism is best understood as a fixation at an early infantile level in which a danger situation is met by refusal to speak.

Morris (1953) described six cases of mutism that were diagnosed through exclusion of hysteria, childhood schizophrenia, hyperkinetic disease, and dementia praecocissima. Morris (1953) reports mainly case history descriptions with common factors including a traumatic situation and a degree of constitutional shyness and timidity. The success of an unspecified "psychiatric" intervention was generally limited, with two cases demonstrating spontaneous recoveries. In two other cases, removal from an environment that was considered the cause of the mutism was met by restoration of speech.

The factors common to the mute children discussed by Salfield et al. (1950) and by Morris (1953) are reported in Table 3.4. Reed (1963) noted that these characteristics were not common to previous work and are nonrepresentative of his cases (see Chapter 5).

Early publication of cases of elective mutism in the American literature also indicated a rapidly growing interest in this area in a number of professional mental health fields (e.g., Adams & Glasner, 1954; Browne et al., 1963; Elson, Pearson, Jones, & Schumacher, 1965; Kass, Gillman, Mattis, Klugman, & Jacobson, 1967; Landgarten, 1975; Parker, Olsen, & Throckmorton, 1960; Pustrom & Speers, 1964; Rigby, 1929; Smayling, 1959; Wright, 1967).

In one of the earliest cases of selective mutism reported in the American literature, Rigby (1929) described a child who at the age of 3½ had given up speech completely. Rigby attributed this problem to "negativism," which she operationalized as not doing something because one is told to do it. The report is generally a discussion of family dynamics and issues purportedly related to the mutism. Although there was no formal treatment program described, the recommendations are quite interesting:

He must be brought to the state where he does as he is told because he is told to do it. The method Dr. Twitmyer recommends for achieving this is "protoplasmic discomfort." Soft words and coaxing may seem to work but they are not the essence of discipline. This boy is too shrewd to be allowed to get away with anything more. Before long, at the rate he is going now, he will run the family out of the house. Spanking is as poor a method as compromise or coaxing. Military discipline is the quickest way to bring him around. He may exhaust the disciplinarian in a few hours but he must be attacked at the moment when he himself is worn

TABLE 3.4*
Factors Common to Elective Mutes as Tabulated by Morris (1953)[a]

| | Cases | | | |
|---|---|---|---|---|
| | V. | B. | D'n. | D'd. |
| Family difficulties (financial) .......................... | − | − | − | − |
| Psychotic or defective heredity ......................... | − | − | − | − |
| Ascertained educationally subnormal .................... | + | − | − | − |
| Disparity in physique ................................... | + | + | − | − |
| Unstable background .................................... | + | − | − | − |
| Delayed milestones (other than speech) ................. | ? | − | ? | − |
| Undue personal timidity................................. | − | + | + | + |
| *Other characteristics* | | | | |
| Incidence of mutism among family or intimates ........... | − | − | − | − |
| Mixed Verbal I.Q. (Terman–Merrill revision of the Binet) .. | 72 | 60 | 61 | 70 |
| Non-Verbal Test I.Q. (Alexander Performance Scale) ...... | 70 | 88 | 60 | 95 |
| Reading Quotients (Schonell Graded Words Test).......... | 49 | 85 | 77 | 101 |
| Arithmetic Quotients (Burt Oral Test) ................... | 54 | 80 | 57 | 88 |
| Age mutism began, according to: Parents ............... | 9 | ?8 | ?2 | 5 |
| Age mutism began, according to: Teachers .............. | 5 | 5 | 5 | 5 |
| Age at referral to clinic .............................. | 13 | 13 | 12 | 12 |
| Report on discharge .................................... | I+ | I | I | N |

+ = Factor present; − = Factor absent.
I+ = Much improved, I = Improved, N = Not improved.
[a]From Reed (1963).

out and there must be no relaxing of the rule. It will be a long task and a hard one, but only when this boy is obedient will he be rescued from imbecility [p. 161].

Adams and Glasner (1954) described four cases of children, but follow-up indicated no progress after leaving the clinic. In yet another case, speech therapy was the primary mode of intervention, with some unspecified concomitant "psychotherapy" offered. The case generally could be considered a failure because after several months of therapy, only several simple words were spoken, and no generalization was programmed. In yet another case, two siblings, ages 9 and 6, were offered speech therapy, the results being met by "resistance" and "hostility." Again, no follow-up measures were reported. Adams and Glasner (1954) stressed the home situation as a primary cause of mutism, noting that children were fearful of fathers who were alcoholic and abusive. In one family, the children were not allowed to make any noise when the father was in a "bad mood." Physical abuse was also apparent. They further noted that the outstanding difference between their cases and those previously discussed in the literature was a strong hostility and resistance to therapy. Interestingly, sign language was sometimes used by the children to communicate.

Browne et al. (1963) reviewed their work with mute children. In one case, after a year and a half of disappointing results, the child was given an injection of desoxy ephedine and amgtal to elicit speech. This procedure was unsuccessful. Browne et al. (1963) also described the case of a boy who, at age 3, first stopped talking to a nurse upon visits to the doctor's office. He then stopped talking to an aunt. Thereafter he became even more selective in his speech, eventually narrowing it to the immediate family, two grandparents, and certain neighborhood children (with adults not present). The child underwent extensive psychotherapy. The authors argued that the mutism could only be understood by studying the entire family constellation and therefore noted that work with the family should be the primary focus of therapy. In this regard, the authors suggested that an improvement in the father correlated with an improvement in the child. In their analysis, mute children are either fixated or regressed to the anal stage; have urinary or bowel difficulty; are shy, negativistic, and withdrawn; regard others as strange or frightening; develop a sadistic relationship toward most adults; and punish people with their mutism.

Elson et al. (1965) reported treatment of four girls (ages 7 to 10 when first seen) and followed them up for 6 months to 6 years, depending on the case. The interventions involved intensive milieu therapy in a residential inpatient treatment center for children. Some features of the follow-up results involved the mothers reporting increased verbalization by the children as a sign of failure of therapy rather than improvement and school attendance at 90% to 100% following discharge; none required further hospitalization or other treatment, and they generally demonstrated good adjustment. Elson et al. (1965) suggested that their cases fell into the category of passive-aggressive personality trait disturbance.

Some writers have documented some success beyond the clinic setting but have failed to establish speech with the therapist (e.g., Chetnik, 1973; Mora, Devault, & Schopler, 1962; Pustrom & Speers, 1964). Chetnik (1973) reported the case of a 6½-year-old child who did not speak to school teachers and peers for a full year. In addition to the mutism, the child displayed numerous fears (e.g., dogs, being alone). The author indicated that conflicts relating to oral, anal, and phallic strivings were worked on during various phases of treatment. Although some forms of communication were observed (e.g., drawing, writing, intense play, body gestures, and some sounds), the child remained silent during the 2-year period of treatment.

Pustrom and Spears (1964) offered a dynamic interpretation of the problem of eliciting speech with the therapist in their treatment of mute children:

> We are concerned that none of these children was able to talk to his therapist even though all were able to talk to others. It is our impression that the child's failure to speak to his therapist represents a last-ditch stand against giving up his omnipotent control of others. One can speculate that as long as this remains, the child, in future stresses, might revert to stubborn silence in dealing with the stress [p. 296].

These authors presented three cases of elective mutism that were diagnosed and treated at the Child Psychiatry Unit of the North Carolina Memorial Hospital. The first child, an 8-year-old boy, was referred because of his refusal to talk in school, stubborn tendencies, disobedience, and enuresis. A second case, also an 8-year-old boy, was referred by a pediatrician because he refused to talk to anyone but a few adults and other children. The third case was an 8-year-old girl who was referred by her parents because of nontalking and social withdrawal. Clinic-based psychotherapy was conducted with the children and their mothers. The focus of therapy with the children was on potentially aggressive impulses and their anticipated consequences and on the dependency relationship with the mothers. The authors found the therapeutic efforts encouraging, even though the children never did speak to their therapist.

Interestingly, some writers viewed the clients' continual refusal to speak, despite therapeutic intervention, an important part of improvement. Mora et al. (1962) reported the case of twin girls referred to school staff because of selective mutism. The girls' mutism was first noted in school when they began subprimary grade at age 5. Attempts by teachers, a counselor, and other guidance staff failed to elicit any verbal response for the following 7 years! Mora et al. (1962) emphasized that the mutism was maintained by "twinship society,"[3] school expectations, and peers. The intervention, conducted by two therapists, first involved breaking the tie of the "twinship" and then encouraging differentiation through talk therapy, drawing, and play therapy. Casework with the mother was also aimed at resolving the ambivalent relationship of twins and mother. The authors reported that the twins developed into more normal socialized patterns during adolescence in that both girls took boyfriends and talked freely with other people. Both children continued to communicate only in writing with the therapists. The authors noted that it provided them with "a means of expressing hostility while maintaining their freedom of self-expression and verbal communication with the rest of the world [p. 51]." The family moved, so that it was impossible to follow up the case (Mora, 1978).

Kass, Gillman, Mattis, Klugman, and Jacobson (1967) reported the case of a 6½-year-old girl who was silent throughout both nursery school and kindergarten. The intervention consisted of individual psychotherapy (unspecified) and integration into a regular first grade, with cooperation and participation from school personnel. The authors claimed success, which was documented through speech in individual sessions, alone with a Braille teacher, and then dramatically during telephone play in the school class. Follow-up indicated that she became a fully integrated class member, and academic achievement was noted as being equal to or surpassing that of her classmates. The cause of mutism was purported to be

---

[3]The "twinship society" refers to a confusion in self-identification of identical twins that causes a delay in normal personality development. It is hypothesized that the "mirror image of the self" serves as a means of mastering their rivalry and reinforces the twinship society sometimes to the point of fantasies of omnipotence.

related to a retentive reaction to trauma, experienced during the anal phase of development, displaced to the oral sphere.

Similar to the formulation offered for school phobia by Leventhal and Sills (1964), Halpern, Hammond, and Cohen (1971) argued that mutism is a speech phobia arising out of an overevaluation by the child of his or her power. The authors review three cases in which the focus of therapy was on eliciting cooperation of school staff to facilitate speech. The first child, age 7, was referred by a public school where he had been totally nonverbal from prekindergarten registration through mid-first-grade. The second two cases were identical twin girls who were referred by the school because they would not speak in first grade, although they talked with both parents, two older brothers, and a younger sister at home. In each case, conferences were scheduled for a discussion of the children, the dynamics of their mutism, tactics to be used in promoting speech, and a contingency program for the teacher. The authors reported generally successful results but no follow-up data.

Laybourne (1979), in his review of elective mutism, presented two case histories that represent examples of psychodynamic interventions. In the first case, a 5-year-old boy was referred to the Division of Child Psychiatry, University of Kansas Medical Center, because he would talk only to family members and close friends of the family. The problem had existed since he was 3. Laybourne noted that although the case was treated before behavior modification became a well-known intervention, this form (i.e., attention getting) of mutism responds best to behavior modification procedures. It was hypothesized that the boy's symptom possibly developed because early in life, his parents thought that his mute behavior was "cute" and reinforced it. Subsequently, the mother was told to tell the child to talk. It was noted that this occurred, and the child did indeed begin to speak to others.

The second case described by Laybourne (1979) represents the "shy, inhibited, schizoid type of child." In such cases, mutism "seems more determined by temperament than by family pathology." The second case that represented an example of the category was a 13-year-old girl who was also referred to the Child Psychiatry Center for a combination of failure to talk in school and extreme negativism. The problem had been evident, in varying degrees, since the age of 6 years. Laybourne describes various therapeutic procedures (some of which involved behavior modification techniques) that were implemented during 10 months of outpatient therapy and during hospitalization on a pediatric ward. Purportedly, the behavior modification procedures only increased her negativism, but a relationship with a floor maid encouraged speaking to nursing staff and child psychiatry personnel. Unfortunately, after discharge from the hospital, she returned home and gradually relapsed into silence at school and in the outpatient setting. A 7-year follow-up revealed that the girl remained silent, speaking only to her parents. Around the age of 20, she was reported to speak in church and other social settings, but she continued shy, reticent, and inhibited behaviors. Laybourne is vehement in indicating that this "type" of child responds poorly to the "mechanistic manipulations of behavior modification."

Adams (1970) presented the case of a 6-year-old boy who had not spoken for 18 months. The child was described as shy, isolated, and passive and currently failing in school due to his mutism. The boy was seen twice a week in psychotherapy (interpreting play and connecting it with past and present conflicts), and his mother was seen for the first 10 minutes of each session. During the first 6 months of therapy, the child did not utter one word. After a total of 14 months of treatment, the child's speech was low and lacked spontaneity, but he would speak to his mother, brother, and sisters. The author attributed the mutism to the mother's abandonment (hospitalization) of him for 10 days with a hostile grandmother who "farmed him out to a neighbor." Accordingly, "this not only activated his basic conflict of fear of loss of love, but accentuated the normal hostility and rivalry operative in any youngster who faces the prospect of being displaced by a new sibling [p. 216]." Although no formal follow-ups are repoted, the author noted that the boy did well in school and became quite verbal.

Psychodynamic therapy has also focused on mutism in adolescents. Kaplan and Escoll (1973) report two case histories of adolescents with initial and prolonged mutism with their therapist. Also, except for an occasional comment, neither had spoken to her family for 1 to 3 years prior to seeking treatment. Both girls were diagnosed as having hysterical personality disorders. The first (Miss Z) was a 15-year-old 10th-grade student who was admitted to a psychiatric inpatient unit with a 9-month history of being bedridden in a succession of general hospitals because of hysterical ataxia following an appendectomy. Following 6 weeks of therapy, Miss Z was reported to be walking, talking, and eating; although she was then discharged to the care of a psychiatrist in her hometown, she had to be readmitted 2 months later with a return of silence and depressive affect. Thereafter, she was hospitalized for 6 months and was again involved in psychotherapy. Presumably, this resulted in improvement, as follow-up by telephone suggested that Miss Z was in school and doing well.

Case 2 (Miss F) was a 17-year-old high school student who had made three suicide attempts in rapid succession. Miss F was admitted to the hospital after 9 months of twice-weekly psychotherapy. During this period, her silence with her therapist was intractable. The present treatment consisted of 30-minute sessions four times per week. After 6 months of treatment, the therapist was transferred. Miss F was reported as talking freely but was depressed.

The authors note that the major dynamics of the two girls were separation, a prohibition against the expression of anger from adolescent to parent, and a sexually stimulating relationship between adolescent patient and father. The initial task was to shift the focus of therapy from the patient's silence to the issue of separation. Although this was accomplished, the results of psychodynamic therapy with these two adolescents were largely a failure.

Ruzicka and Sackin (1974) take a somewhat different perspective in their presentation of a case of selective mutism. They discuss the implications of the mutism on the therapist in light of previous discussions of patient silence during psychoanalytic psychotherapy (e.g., Blos, 1972; Fliess, 1949; Weisman, 1955; Zeligs, 1961). Their report is a description of the therapist's (Mrs. Ruzicka) "feelings" during the course of individual psychotherapy with a 9-year-old girl who demonstrated selective mutism. After several months of therapy, the authors noted that the child became more relaxed and demonstrated enjoyment during game play. A major point made by the authors is that painful tensions created during silent periods, if allowed to remain in the therapist's unconscious, can lead to lapses in empathy and to impulsive, destructive interventions. Presumably, in the present report, the therapist was able to work through these concerns. The authors raised three concerns that they believe must be considered by anyone who undertakes individual psychoanalytic therapy with a mute child:

1. The mute patient always evokes specific, intense, and usually distressing responses in the therapist.
2. These responses are an invaluable source of information about the patient's inner state; in effect, whatever the patient may be experiencing is communicated to the therapist, not through words, but through those affects and fantasies stimulated in the therapist by the patient's behavior. Therefore, it is essential that the therapist be constantly attuned to his own thoughts and feelings, while simultaneously remaining alert to the more direct modes of nonverbal communication as conveyed through the patient's behavior.
3. The therapist's effective utilization of these communications will enable him to remain empathetically tuned to his patient: thereby apparent stalemates may be avoided, and impulsive interventions, motivated by the therapist's helplessness and frustration, may be forestalled [p. 560].

## Dynamic Speech Therapy Approaches

In some respects, it is unusual that more reports of selective mutism have not been reported in the speech literature (e.g., as reflected in the *Journal of Speech and Hearing Disorders*). Nevertheless, several studies have been reported in this area. Strait (1958) did not label her case "elective" mutism, but rather described a child who was "speechless in school and social life" but who exhibited normal speech in the family unit. Therapy consisted of a series of speech sessions in which the therapist talked with the child, encouraged reading, and involved him in social situations. The involvement continued for several months, and success was reported.

Smayling (1959) reported the analysis of six cases of "voluntary mutism" in children ranging in age from 5½ to 10 years who were referred to a clinic facility. All cases were seen for two or three individual, half-hour speech therapy periods weekly. In each case, the child's mother observed a minimum of one training period each month and was generally present in the training room for each period. The speech therapy focused on correction of speech and language behavior utilizing conventional speech training methods, but no attempt was made to alleviate the mutism per se. Although Smagling (1959) notes that speech therapy was the primary therapeutic variable accounting for success in some cases, considerable influence may have occurred because of some unspecified psychiatric intervention either prior to or during the speech intervention. Various operant reinforcement and modification of vegetative and respiratory reflexes subserving speech were employed. Case A began speaking in the classroom and in all other situations immediately after her sixth speech session, and no reversion to mutism occurred. Cases B and C (twin girls) were observed to have no mutism at the end of 3 months of therapy. Case D was reported to show signs of "psychological disturbances" and was engaged in both speech therapy and some unspecified psychiatric treatment carried out twice a week. Although Smagling (1959) reported that within 2 months, the mutism in all situations was absent, the contribution of the psychiatric intervention is unknown. Treatment of Case E, who also experienced an articulation problem, was unsuccessful despite concomitant psychiatric intervention (unspecified). The child, who had completed her kindergarten year at the initiation of therapy, remained mute through the fourth grade. Case F was involved in psychiatric treatment (unspecified) for more than 2 years with no apparent results and was then discontinued. After initiation of speech therapy, the child responded consistently to all stimuli, but all responses were whispered, and no voicing occurred. Subsequently, after a 21-month period, normal speech patterns developed in the speech sessions and were reported to have generalized to the school. Smayling (1959) argued that speech therapy techniques that do not include psychotherapy or play therapy seem advisable for cases with genuine language and speech defects.

## Dynamic Art Therapy Interventions

There have been relatively few reported cases where art therapy has been the primary mode of treatment for the selective mute (e.g., Howard, 1963; Landgarten, 1975), although it has been used as a supplement to other conventional forms of psychotherapy discussed earlier (e.g., Chetnik, 1973; Heuger & Morgenstern, 1927; Mora et al., 1962). Landgarten (1978) noted that she has worked with more than 15 cases of elective mutism. Howard (1963) reported the case of an 8-year-old child who was referred to a hospital for not talking in school, but who was quite talkative at home. The child was diagnosed as "psychoneurotic, anxiety reaction." During the first 6 months, daily art therapy progressed through five phases: passive, fantasy, oedipal anxiety, aggressive, and again a passive stage. Eventually, the child was withdrawn from therapy but still remained mute at school.

Landgarten (1975) presented the case of a 7-year-old girl referred to an outpatient clinic because she refused to talk. Art sessions were scheduled wherein the child and sometimes her siblings were required to paint. The author reports that initially, children were given cookies and candy somewhat randomly, whereas later, candy was given contingently on painting. The author reports that the 7-month art therapy was generally successful. However, a follow-up after 4 months indicated a regression to nonspeaking, presumably due to the abandonment of the family. However, more recent information on the former client suggests that she demonstrates functional speech but exhibits "shy" behavior (Landgarten, 1978).

## SUMMARY OF PSYCHODYNAMIC INTERVENTIONS

More than 20 reports of description and/or treatment of selective mutism have been reported in the psychodynamic literature. Psychoanalytic research has discussed the close relation between mutism and the mother–child interaction. In this regard, many writers have reported early disturbances and fixations at preoedipal levels. Laybourne ( 1979 ) observed that there is some evidence of a fixation at the anal stage of development but that other developmental tasks are also involved.

Although quite diverse therapeutic interventions have been employed with mute children, it remains difficult to specify the therapeutic mechanisms because of the lack of clear operational definitions of terms and little if any data on therapeutic effectiveness. Generally, the majority of writers report successful interventions. Writers using "speech therapy" interventions generally show a positive pattern of results, but again it remains questionable as to what specific therapeutic mechanisms were operating. Unsuccessful reports are characteristic of the art therapy approaches, but some unpublished data suggest some positive outcomes. Nevertheless, a major problem with the psychodynamic interventions is that many procedures were used simultaneously, often by many different therapists who used different techniques.

Generally, a consistent theme running throughout the psychodynamic literature is that this childhood problem is difficult to treat. This is reflected in the overall length of the treatment period (e.g., several months to several years), the lack of consistent generalization from the treatment setting (predominately in the clinic setting) to other areas in the natural environment where the mutism occurred (e.g., school), and the lack of consistent follow-up and no maintenance when follow-up assessment did occur.

# 4 Behavior Modification: A Perspective

This chapter is intended to provide a general overview of current issues in behavior modification, particularly its use in applied settings. There are literally hundreds of texts dealing with various aspects of behavior modification, and the interested reader is referred to some primary sources for a comprehensive overview (Bandura, 1969; Catania & Brigham, 1978; Craighead, Kazdin, & Mahoney, 1976; Gelfand & Hartmann, 1975; Kazdin, 1980a; Marholin, 1978; Sulzer-Azaroff & Mayer, 1977). This chapter is primarily designed to elucidate certain features of the behavioral approach that help set it apart from the psychodynamic view discussed in Chapter 2. It does not deal with critical issues in the area of controversy or attempt to embrace the many new dimensions of behavior modificaion such as the use of cognitive therapeutic procedures (e.g., Meichenbaum, 1977) and self-control techniques (e.g., Mahoney & Thoresen, 1974; Thoresen & Mahoney, 1974).

## SCOPE OF BEHAVIOR MODIFICATION

It is useful to clarify the relation between behavior modification and the broader concept of behavior influence. Stolz, Wienchowski, and Brown (1975) contrasted these two concepts by suggesting that whereas behavior influence occurs whenever one person exerts some degree of control over another (e.g., formal education, child rearing, interpersonal interactions), behavior modification refers to a special form of behavior influence that involves the application of principles derived from research in experimental psychology to alleviate human suffering and enhance human functioning (p. 1027). In many respects, the behavioral model of deviant behavior that developed out of psychological research helped to provide an identity to psychology independent of medicine where psychodynamic approaches were closely aligned. In addition to providing a unique perspective in the treatment of deviant behavior, the behavioral approach provided an important alternative to the disease model of deviant behavior (as outlined in Chapter 2 and demonstrated in one area of child practice in Chapter 3). Thus, in many ways, the traditional intrapsychic-disease model and an accompanying dissatisfaction with it provided the context from which behavior modification developed (Kazdin, 1978a).An excellent account of the history of behavior modification as well as current-day perspectives in the field has been provided by Kazdin (1978a), and the interested reader is referred to this source.

Current-day behavior modification procedures and approaches are quite diverse, making it difficult to define the field clearly. Kazdin and Wilson (1978) discussed five different conceptual schemes that can be included in contemporary behavior modification. These include applied behavior analysis, a neobehavioristic mediational model, social learning theory, cognitive behavior modification, and multimodel behavior therapy. Multimodel behavior therapy (cf. Lazarus, 1977) is sometimes not included within the behavior therapy conceptualization. Applied behavior analysis is defined broadly as the application of interventions to alter behaviors of clinical and social importance (Baer, Wolf, & Risley, 1968). The neobehavioristic, mediational S–R model is generally defined as the application of the principles of conditioning, especially classical conditioning and counterconditioning, to the treatment of deviant behavior. Practice in this area derives from the work of such individuals as Eysenck (1960, 1964), Rachman (1963), and Wolpe (1958). The social learning conceptualization of behavior therapy represents a comprehensive approach to human behavior in which both normal and deviant functioning is assumed to be developed and maintained on the basis of three distinct regulatory systems (Bandura, 1977b). Finally, the cognitive behavior modification approach (e.g., Mahoney, 1974; Mahoney & Arnkoff, 1978; Meichenbaum, 1974, 1977) incorporates a number of diverse therapeutic procedures. A major feature of cognitive behavior therapy is its emphasis on the importance of cognitive processes and private events as mediators of behavior change (cf. Kazdin & Wilson, 1978, pp. 1–7).

Likely, more diversity will characterize the future of behavior modification, particularly with the "cognitive drift" that is occurring in some areas of the field. Nevertheless, there are some general characteristics that have wide acceptance and that can be subsumed under the rubric of behavior modification (Kazdin, 1978):

1. Focus upon current rather than historical determinants of behavior;
2. Emphasis on overt behavior change as the main criterion by which treatment should be evaluated;
3. Specification of treatment in objective terms so as to make replication possible;

4. Reliance upon basic research in psychology as a source of hypotheses about treatment and specific therapy techniques; and

5. Specificity in defining, treating, and measuring the target problems in therapy [p. 375].

Generally, these assumptions represent a rejection of certain aspects of the intrapsychic-disease view of abnormal behavior and an embracing of a scientific approach toward treatment and practice.

## GENERAL CHARACTERISTICS OF THE BEHAVIORAL APPROACH

The aforementioned characteristics suggest that there are some unifying features of the behavior modification approach despite apparent diversity. I now describe in more detail some features of the behavior modification approach that set it apart from the psychodynamic approaches discussed in Chapter 2. These include the behavioral views of abnormal behavior, emphases on experimental research findings, direct focus on behavior, methodology, and the behavioral focus of diagnosis, assessment, and treatment.

### The Behavioral Approach Toward Abnormal Behavior

The behavioral model of deviant behavior posits that psychopathology is mainly a set of learned maladaptive behaviors rather than the product of physical disease or inferred motives, needs, impulses, and drives, which are hypothesized to direct behavior. In the behavioral approach, an emphasis is placed upon environmental, situational, and social influences that direct behavior.

In this conceptualization, abnormal behavior is perceived as indistinct from normal behavior in terms of its development. Of course, there are exceptions to this position, as in the case where definite brain pathology, physical disease, and drug-induced states are apparent. Nevertheless, most deviant behavior is not represented as a disease process. Rather, behavior treatment within the behavioral model involves applying specific procedures from established principles of learning to change maladaptive behavior and to facilitate the acquisition of desirable adaptive behavior patterns. Certain principles of learning are used to explain behavior irrespective of whether it can be labeled as deviant.

Within the behavioral model, it is generally recognized that the labeling of behavior as abnormal or deviant is based on subjective judgments rather than objective criteria (Bandura, 1969; Kazdin, 1975; Szasz, 1960; Ullmann & Krasner, 1969). Within this context, certain behaviors may be viewed differently in individuals as deviant or normal. Children who are brought to the attention of professionals represent a highly selective, biased sample of those who manifest a given behavior (Ross, 1974). Moreover, the prevalence of the kind of behavior that brings children to the attention of relevant clinics and agencies has been demonstrated in unselected samples of the "normal" population (e.g., Conners, 1970; Lapoure & Mouk, 1959, 1964; Werr & Quay, 1971). In this regard, selective mutism is likely of much higher incidence than the literature reflects. Many cases may not be brought to the attention of professionals because it is labeled as acceptable from the parents' standpoint. A teacher may view a silent child as an especially desirable student among a group of generally talkative, first-grade children. In contrast, the perception of the school psychologist or counselor may be radically different. He or she may perceive a problem in a child who speaks only in select settings or only to certain individuals. Thus, the individual who evaluates a particular behavior has a major role in determining whether it is labeled normal or abnormal.

In the case of children demonstrating mute behavior in select stimulus settings, the social context is important in determining whether the behavior can be regarded as deviant. Typically, such behavior could be evaluated against social norms. Deviant behavior is often inferred from the degree to which the behavior deviates from social norms (cf. Scheff, 1973). However, because social norms can vary considerably across different cultural groups, it is sometimes difficult to provide an objective criterion for deviant behavior. A behavior therapist might find it difficult to convince parents that their child's mute behavior is deviant if they operate from the child-rearing philosophy that "children should be seen but not heard." Nevertheless, the labeling of the behavior as deviant by the therapist is based on subjective value judgments rather than on evidence of maladaptive or diseased psychological processes. Thus, the differences in behavior across individuals reflect differences on the same continuum rather than differences in qualitative illness and health (Kazdin, 1975).

In recent years, applied behavioral researchers have increasingly been concerned with determining the clinical importance of behavior change. This process involves a procedure called *social validation* (cf. Kazdin, 1977b; Wolf, 1978). Within the context of focusing on behavior change, social validation refers to assessing the social acceptability of intervention programs. Kazdin (1977b) lists some facets of the acceptability process. First, the acceptability of the *focus* of the intervention can be evaluated. This aspect refers to whether the behaviors selected are important to individuals in the natural environment. In addition to the focus of the intervention, the acceptability of the *procedures* can be assessed. Consumer satisfaction with a procedure (e.g., reinforcement, time-out) can be determined and used as a basis for selecting among effective techniques. The final facet involves as assessment of the importance of the *behavior change* achieved with treatment. This is validated by examining the change in light of the performance of nondeviant peers in the environment or through evaluations by individuals in routine contact with the client.

To determine whether behavior change is clinically important for the client, validation of the intervention effect is necessary. Validation of the intervention effect is accomplished through *social comparison* and *subjective evaluation* methods (Kazdin, 1977b). In the social comparison method, an essential feature of the process is to compare the behavior of the client before and after treatment with the behavior of "nondeviant" peers. This procedure asks the question: "Is the client's behavior after treatment distinguishable from the behavior of peers?" For example, one might compare the formerly mute child's new level of speech to that of peers in the classroom. Subjective evaluation involves an evaluation of the client's behavior by individuals who are in common contact with him or her to determine whether the change made during treatment is important. This procedure asks the question: "Has the behavior change led to qualitative differences in how the client is viewed by others?" For example, judgments by teachers, parents, or other socialization agents could be obtained to determine how they view the results of the treatment program.

Although social validation procedures represent an important advance in evaluation of therapeutic outcomes, it still remains as a somewhat subjective process. Normative standards may be perceived as an inappropriate standard against which to evaluate change; normative groups may be difficult to determine for some individuals; and persons conducting the subjective evaluations may not establish consistent criteria or may not perceive clinically significant changes in line with the behavior therapist; and/or various rating scales employed to make these judgments may lack reliability and validity. A major concern with social validation is that the subjective nature of the criterion leaves the level of performance needed for clinical change somewhat unspecified. Needless to say, employing social validation procedures suggests that there is a recognition of the need to consider deviant behavior in a social context and to promote consideration of multiple evaluation criteria on both focus and outcome measures.

## Focus on Direct Measurement of Behavior

Traditional approaches to the understanding and treatment of deviant behavior have used indirect measurement systems to find the causes of problems. It is commonly assumed that test responses within the indirect measurement approach are signs of enduring personality traits or states that are evidence across diverse situations (cf. Tryon, 1979). Tests are administered to obtain information about certain forces that direct personality and rarely are examined in terms of overt qualities (Herson & Barlow, 1976). This indirect form of assessment has been labeled the "indirect-sign paradigm" by Mischel (1972). He indicates:

> It is usually assumed that the person's underlying dispositions are relatively generalized and will manifest themselves pervasively in diverse aspects of his behavior, especially when the situation is unstructured and ambiguous and the

examiner's purpose is disguised, as in projective testing. Motives, needs, psychodynamics, complexes, basic attitudes, and other psychic forces are hypothesized as the underlying but not direct observable dispositions that generate numerous diverse manifestations, much as physical disease produces a host of clinical symptoms [p. 319].

Thus, the indirect assessment approach characteristic of many traditional prardigms (such as the psychodynamic model discussed in Chapter 2) considers various behaviors as signs of some underlying process.

In contrast to indirect measurement approaches, a response obtained through direct measurement in the behavioral approach is viewed as a sample of a larger population of similar responses elicited under particular stimulus conditions (Mischel, 1972). The most common, direct measurement techniques include motoric, self-report (or cognitive), and physiological (see following discussion on assessment). Direct observations of clients in natural settings (e.g., classroom, home) have been the common form of direct measurement procedures. When naturalistic observation is not possible or feasible, analogue situations that approximate the more natural environment can be employed (e.g., Nay, 1977). Self-reports may also be employed on occasion, but it is assumed that such verbal responses may operate under different contingencies than the actual behavioral referent.

In recent years, there has been more diversity in the measures that are used in direct measurement. Many behavioral psychologists consider that cognitions, feelings, and so forth should be included in direct measurements of a client. Physiological response systems (e.g., muscle tension, heart rate, blood pressure, respiration) have also been included in direct measurement systems. Hersen and Barlow (1976) have provided an overview of these measurement systems and the interrelations among them. Is should also be emphasized that some behavior therapists suggest that private events (thoughts) mediate problematic behavior and are targeted for treatment. Other therapists (e.g., applied behavior analysts) eschew virtually all mediational states and prefer rather to focus on overt behavior and the external environment (Kazdin, 1978a).

A number of advantages can be identified when direct measurement procedures are employed (cf. Hersen & Barlow, 1976). First, complex interpretations involving a complex network of theoretical structures are not required. Second, predictive validity increases as the discrepancy is diminished between the behavior sampled and the behavior that is predicted (of course, sampled behaviors and the predicted behaviors are the same when observations are made in a naturalistic setting where the problem occurs). Third, when using direct measurement techniques, there is a close relation between target behaviors selected for modification and the actual treatment process (see later section on assessment).

### Experimenal Research Base

A major contribution of the behavioral approach to solving applied problems is a knowledge base that can be used in the design of intervention plans. It is a basic premise of behavior therapy that the scientific method should be used to discover, describe, and utilize lawful relationships between behavior and its determinants (Ross & Nelson, 1979). Behavior modification techniques grew from diverse areas and techniques of psychological research. Today, behavioral research covers a large domain including basic and applied investigation. Yates (1970) provided a definition of behavior modification that reflects its diversity in using a variety of theories and empirical findings:

> Behavior therapy is the attempt to utilize systematically that body of empirical and theoretical knowledge which has resulted from the application of the experimental method in psychology and its closely related disciplines (physiology and neurophysiology) in order to explain the genesis and maintenance of abnormal patterns of behavior; and to apply that knowledge to the treatment or prevention of those abnormalities by means of controlled experimental studies of the single case, both descriptive and remedial [p. 18].

Use of the behavioral knowledge base in the design of interventions has the important advantage of producing plans based on principles that have been found to be effective in controlled research. Interventions based on empirical research should have a greater probability of success than programs derived from informal sources of information such as clinical experience (cf. Bergan, 1977).

*Methodology.*   An important contribution of behavior modification is that it offers a means of assessment of behavior and experimental evaluation of interventions. Generally, behavior modification has developed within a tradition of experimentation and evaluation (Kazdin, 1978a; Kazdin & Marholin, 1978). Some writers have argued that a data-oriented methodology should be the basis for the treatment of deviant behavior, just as the scientist-practitioner method should guide the therapist in clinical practice (cf. Browning & Stover, 1971; Wetzel, Balch, & Kratochwill, 1979).

The behavioral-analytic approach has been a prominent means of evaluating treatment plans. This approach, referred to as the functional analysis of behavior, is summarized by Peterson (1968):

> The central features of the method are (1) systematic observation of the problem behavior to obtain a response frequency baseline, (2) systematic observation of the stimulus conditions following and/or preceding the behavior, with special concern for antecedent discriminative cues and consequent reinforcers, (3) experimental manipulation of a condition which is functionally, hence causally, related to the

problem behavior, and (4) further observation to record any changes in behavior which may occur [p. 114].

In recent years the behavior modification field has been characterized by a great deal of diversity in research approaches (Kratochwill & Brody, 1978; O'Leary & Kent, 1973). The more strict operant approach to treatment has been characterized by the single-subject research strategy, but even here diversity in methodology is increasingly becoming a characteristic of the area (Kazdin, 1975). There is a variety of different experimental designs that can be used to evaluate a behavior modification program. Detailed discussions of various designs and accompanying methodological issues in behavior modification are provided in other sources (cf. Bailey, 1977; Hersen & Barlow, 1976; Kazdin, 1980a; Kratochwill, 1978; Sidman, 1960; Thoresen, in press). Issues relating to single-subject research are also discussed in more detail in Chapter 6 of this volume.

Several positive features of a data-based approach to therapeutic efforts can be listed (Wetzel et al., 1979). First, data evaluation provides the behavior therapist with client feedback about behaviors in a particular environment and the relation between these target behaviors and individuals who may be maintaining the behaviors. Second, the data-gathering activities of significant others in the client's environment can also be used as a source of feedback to demonstrate how their behavior influences client behavior. Finally, actual change in the client's behavior is documented and can be shared with other professionals and individuals responsible for the welfare of the child.

## Behavioral Diagnosis

Some specific features of behavioral approaches to diagnosis and classification were detailed in Chapter 1, and so only some general characteristics are reviewed here.

A general purpose of behavioral diagnosis is the identification of target behaviors that need to be changed and the environmental events that influence behavior. Nevertheless, recommendations for behavioral approaches to classification (Cautela & Upper, 1973; Goldfried & Pomeranz, 1968; Kanfer & Saslow, 1965, 1969; Mischel, 1968;) have evolved because of perceived weaknesses in conventional psychiatric systems (e.g., DSM-II) and the debatable metapsychological assumptions their use involves (Begelman, 1976). But as Kazdin (1978a) has noted, no concrete system of behavioral diagnosis tends to be followed in practice. Behavior therapists typically discuss general classes of behavioral problems in terms of behavioral assets, deficits, excesses, and so forth (cf. Bijou & Grimm, 1975; Marholin, & Bijou, 1978; Bijou & Peterson, 1971; Goldfried & Davidson, 1976; Kanfer & Saslow, 1969; Krasner & Ullmann, 1973). For example, Goldfried and Davidson (1976), in outlining various categories of deviant behaviors, suggest taking into account stimulus as well as client variables and further categorize deviant behaviors according to the variables that possibly maintain them. These general categories include: (1) difficulties in stimulus control of behavior (e.g., defective stimulus control, inappropriate stimulus control); (2) deficient behavioral repertoires; (3) aversive behavioral repertoires; (4) difficulties with incentive (reinforcer) systems (e.g., defective incentive system in the individual, inappropriate incentive system in the individual, absence of incentives in the environment); and (5) aversive self-reinforcing systems (pp. 28–32).

It is important to emphasize that behavioral diagnosis is closely linked to assessment. Generally, a behavior therapist conducting a behavioral analysis would first determine what brought the client to the attention of the therapist (Ullman & Krasner, 1969). One major purpose of behavioral diagnosis is to reformulate the client's problem in behavioral terms. The reformulation of various problems in behavioral terms helps to identify specific response units so that behavior and any subsequent change can be viewed more analytically than occurs when global descriptions are used to describe clinical problems (Kazdin, 1978a). Following a specific identification of the target behaviors, the conditions under which the behavior(s) occur(s) or do(es) not occur are evaluated. An analysis of the events that precede and follow the activity is typically included. A treatment typically follows this sequence of events.

## Behavioral Assessment

Although behavioral assessment has been a concern among numerous behavioral investigators (e.g., Bandura, 1969; Goldfried & Kent, 1972; Goldfried & Pomeranz, 1968; Goldfried & Sprafkin, 1974; Kanfer & Phillips, 1970; Kanfer & Saslow, 1969; Mischel, 1968; Stuart, 1970), it is only recently that the topic has been given increased attention (e.g., Ciminero, Calhoun, & Adams, 1977; Hersen & Barlow, 1976; Hersen & Bellack, 1976; Kratochwill, 1981; Marholin, 1978; O'Leary & Johnson, 1979). In this section, I: (1) review some general differences between behavioral and traditional assessment; (2) discuss some various models of assessment; and (3) review some general assessment methods.

*Behavioral and traditional assessment.*    All assessment practices share the common goal of obtaining reliable and valid information, but a great deal of diversity exists over what the most useful method is. There are several differences between behavioral and traditional (psychodynamic) assessment that can be detailed (Ciminero et al., 1977; Goldfried & Kent, 1972; Herson, 1976). One of the first differences relates to the repeated-measures strategy employed in assessment. Behavioral assessment is frequently characterized by some form of continuous measurement of a target behavior over the duration of the treatment program (Hersen & Barlow, 1976). This form of assessment is possibly more common in the applied behavior analysis area than in other areas of behavior therapy. Nevertheless, the repeated-assessment strategy typically contrasts with traditional assessment wherein the client is assessed on a battery of tests prior to (and sometimes following) a therapeutic program. Moreover, as already noted, *direct* assessment measures are usually preferred over indirect strategies such as projective tests.

A second difference relates to general conceptions of personality held by the behavioral and traditional assessor. Both state (dynamic) and trait (psychometric) approaches infer some underlying constructs that account for consistency in an individual's behavior. Assessment is therefore viewed as a sign of constructs that have presumed relevance in the prediction of behavior. In contrast, the behavioral approach is less inferential in postulating constructs to account for behavior. Goldfried and Kent (1972) note:

> Whereas traditional tests of personality involve the assessment of hypothesized personality constructs which, in turn, are used to predict overt behavior, the behavioral approach entails more of a direct sampling of the criterion behaviors themselves. In addition to requiring fewer inferences than traditional tests, behavioral assessment procedures are seen as being based on assumptions more amenable to direct empirical test and more consistent with empirical evidence [p. 409].

Another important difference between behavioral and traditional assessment relates to the selection of test items and/or situations for assessment. In traditional assessment, items are chosen under the assumption that pathology generally remains stable across situations. Thus, the same test content is used regardless of the situation. Moreover, test content is often disguised by making the items ambiguous. The behavior assessment strategy focuses on the specific relation between certain target behaviors and environments in which the behaviors occur or do not occur. Therefore, there is typically a systematic attempt to sample these situations adequately. Direct observation has been a primary means of assessment, with methods of observation varying depending on specific target problems and intervention programs (Cone & Hawkins, 1977; Hersen & Bellack, 1976; Marholin, 1978).

Earlier it was mentioned that there is a close relation between diagnosis, assessment, and treatment in the behavioral model. This relation between assessment and treatment represents a fourth major difference between behavioral and traditional assessment. Stuart (1970) noted that diagnosis resulting from traditional assessment methods does not accurately predict what treatment should be implemented. The behavioral approach has a direct relation to treatment. Two aims of behavioral assessment are the selection of a treatment technique and the subsequent evaluation of the intervention program (Ciminero et al., 1977). Thus, assessment is conceptualized as part of treatment and is ongoing with treatment.

*Models of behavioral assessment.* Ciminero (1977) lists three major functions of behavioral assessment: (1)*description* of the problem; (2) *selection* of a treatment strategy; and (3) *evaluation* of the treatment outcome.

In behavior modification, treatment is closely aligned with assessment. Whereas treatment focuses directly on problematic behaviors that are targeted, there is no general model that assists in selecting an appropriate strategy (Ciminero, 1977). Presumably, there should be some relation between the treatment technique and the response mode assessed. However, efforts to find these correct "matches" are just beginning.

Recently, Cone (1978) has proposed a conceptual framework for behavioral assessment. In behavioral assessment, three different content areas (Cone, 1977), systems (Hersen & Barlow, 1976; Lang, 1968, 1971, 1977), or channels (Paul & Berstein, 1973) are included—namely, motor, cognitive (self-report), and physiological. Generally, motor content includes activities that involve striate musculature typically observable without instrumentation (e.g., walking, hitting). Physiological contents include activities of muscles and glands that are anatomically innervated and tonic muscle activity (e.g., heart rate, galvanic skin response). Although cognitive activities are not easily defined, Cone (1978) suggested that verbal and cognitive behaviors not be treated as synonymous. Thus, whereas the *act* of speaking is motoric, the referents of speech may be cognitive, motor, or physiological.

A second dimension offered by Cone (1978) involves the various methods that can be used to assess the three aforementioned systems. These dimensions include indirect (i.e., interview, self-report, rating by others) and direct (i.e., self-observation, analog: role play, analog: free behavior, naturalistic: role play, and naturalistic: free behavior). Interviews and self-reports represent an indirect end of the continuum, because behavior observed using these methods is a verbal representation of certain activities taking place at some other time and place. Likewise, ratings by others represent an indirect category because such assessment represents retrospective descriptions.

Direct observation methods are separated into five types, depending on: (1) who is observing; (2) the instructions given the observer; and (3) when the observation occurs. Self-observation or self-monitoring refers to the observation of some important behavior when it occurs. Analogue situations refer to settings or situations that are analogous to, but not the same as, the natural environment (e.g., a clinic office). This type of method can be role played or free to vary. Finally, naturalistic environmental assessment can be used in which behavior is either role played or free to vary.

Figure 4.1 shows that when the content and method dimensions are juxtaposed, a $3 \times 8 = 24$-category, taxonomic system results. Thus, the three content areas are assumed to be measurable through each of the eight methods. For example, measurement of a child's frequency of verbalizations (motor behavioral content) may occur in the natural environment (home and school).

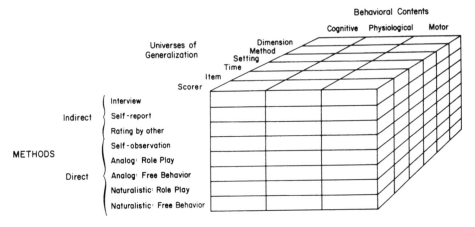

BEHAVIORAL ASSESSMENT GRID

FIG. 4.1.   The Behavioral Assessment Grid (BAG)—a taxonomy of behavioral assessment integrating contents, methods, and universes of generalization. (Source: Cone, J. D. The Behavioral Assessment Grid (BAG): A conceptual framework and a taxonomy. *Behavior Therapy*, 1978, 9, 882–888. Reproduced by permission of Academic Press and the author.)

Cone (1978) has noted too that the behavioral assessor may also be concerned with generalization across six universes: (1) score, (2) item, (3) time, (4) setting, (5) method, and (6) dimension (see Cone, 1977, for a more thorough discussion of this generalization scheme). This final component allows the researcher/assessor to classify a particular measure on the types of generalizability that have been established for it.

The Behavioral Assessment Grid (BAG) has several advantages in future behavioral assessment work. First, it provides a conceptual scheme for organizing behavioral assessment procedures and measures. Second, it provides a scheme for research on behavioral assessment procedures, particularly the interrelationships among various measures (e.g., self-report and direct observation). Third, as new behavioral assessments are developed, they can be assigned to categories in the BAG, allowing more easy selection by researchers and practitioners. Finally, the BAG may contribute to standardization efforts in behavioral assessment.

It is beyond the scope of this chapter to deal with the many treatment strategies that have evolved from the behavior modification model. Suffice it to say that the field is actually evolving in a direction that includes treatment techniques that extend beyond the operant approach. For example, such procedures as systematic desensitization, aversion therapy, flooding and implosion, covert conditioning, modeling, biofeedback, and cognitive techniques are commonly employed in behavior therapy. Most of the therapeutic procedures employed in the treatment of selective mutism stem from the operant model (see

Chapter 4). Some of the operant interventions are discussed in more detail in Chapter 7. A detailed account of the many operant procedures employed in applied settings can be found in several sources (e.g., Bandura, 1969; Kazdin, 1978 a, 1980a; Sulzer-Azaroff & Mayer, 1977).

## SUMMARY AND CONCLUSIONS

Behavior therapy procedures are actively evolving. While early developments in behavior modification were tied to learning theory, the current focus appears to be on establishing behavior change techniques with an empirical research base, but independent of specific theoretical paradigms (see Kazdin, 1978). Contemporary conceptualizations of behavior therapy include applied behavior analysis, the neobehavioristic mediational S-R model, social learning theory, and cognitive behavior modification. This means that assessment and treatment procedures encompass a wide range of techniques. Yet despite this apparent diversity, some general features characterize the field. These include a focus on current rather than historical influence on behavior, an emphasis on overt behavior change to evaluate treatment outcomes, objective specification of the presenting problem, reliance on basic research to develop treatment procedures, and specificity in defining, treating, and measuring problem behaviors.

# 5 Behavioral Research on Selective Mutism

The evolution of behavior modification procedures toward the solution of applied problems has provided a revolution in psychological treatment of deviant behavior. The application of behavioral procedures, particularly applied behavior analysis, to the treatment of childhood selective mutism has steadily increased over the past 15 years (cf. Kratochwill et al., 1979). In many respects, an examination of the behavioral procedures applied to selective mutism reflects the evolution of behavioral treatment procedures, particularly in the area of methodology. Nevertheless, treatment procedures for selective mutism remain closely tied to operant strategies, just as they have been in the behavioral treatment of nonlanguage children (cf. Harris, 1975).

The behavioral literature on selective mutism can be dissected in several ways. In this chapter, I have chosen to discuss the various interventions in terms of methodological approach (case study vs. some formal single-case design). This approach (also taken by the author and his colleagues in previous work [cf. Kratochwill et al., 1979]) is purely arbitrary, because one of several categorical schemes could be employed (e.g., setting, treatment technique, and so forth). Generally, the behavioral literature can be segmented into investigations using retrospective evaluations, case studies, and those using some type of formal research design.

## NONTREATMENT REPORTS

Like some reports in the psychodynamic literature, the behavioral literature contains a retrospective evaluation of clinic cases and an attempt to provide classification and treatment strategies.

Friedman and Karagan (1973) saw 13 mute children at the psychological diagnostic clinic at the University of Iowa. The referral of all the children to the clinic related to school functioning in that all were in their first or second year of school and were described by their teachers as mute. Based on these cases, the authors suggested (1973) that mute children can generally be divided into two groups:

The first group appears to use refusal to speak in a coercive fashion in order to manipulate the immediate environment. In the other group, it appears that speaking is sufficiently anxiety producing so that the child chooses to remain mute. It has been suggested that the reduction in anxiety that results from mute behavior serves as a reward and reinforces the act of remaining mute. Characteristically, these children are described by their parents, teachers, and friends as shy and socially inept [p. 250].

The authors argued that the nonverbal behavior of the mute child is learned and occurs in response to anxiety and fear. As such, they drew a direct parallel between mute children and Dollard and Miller's (1950) discussion of mutism that develops under conditions of extreme stress (e.g., combat anxiety). Conceptualization of mutism as a learned behavior led Friedman and Karagan (1973) to offer seven procedures for management of these children:

1. Individuals treating mute children should avoid coercive practices to force the child to speak. The use of incentives is considered inappropriate because these tactics undermine the child's security and increase anxiety.
2. The child should be included in peer activities at home and in school.
3. Individuals in contact with the child should stress verbal activities, but only under comfortable conditions.
4. Parents should encourage visits with relatives in order that the child will speak in their presence.
5. The child should be encouraged in nonverbal, nonthreatening, interpersonal relationships with adults at school and in the home.
6. Once an adequate relationship has been established between a teacher and the child, an initial attempt should be made to encourage speech. The child should be asked simple questions that necessitate only simple answers of a single word or two. This program should be repeated within the classroom with the child's verbal behavior continuing in all one-to-one situations.
7. The child and all socialization agents in whose presence the child will speak should be encouraged to participate in activities outside the home and in the presence of people who are strangers to the child [pp. 250–252].

Many of these suggestions by Friedman and Karagan (1973) presumably offer useful strategies for intervention with mute children. In their sample of 13 seen at University of Iowa clinics, all continued in school; all referral sources noted continued improvement in the children; and no subsequent referrals were made because of further management problems.

Nonetheless, it appears premature to group children into different categories based on the limited sample size of 13. Moreover, many of the aforementioned suggestions for management of mutism are not empirically documented and should be used with caution. Further discussion of these issues is provided in Chapter 7.

## CASE STUDY INVESTIGATIONS

Case study methodology represented, with few exceptions, the sole methodology of clinical investigation through the first half of the 20th century (Hersen & Barlow, 1976). The case study method provided the clinical base for many single-case investigations of selective mutism. Even some of the more recent reports in the behavioral literature contain this form of methodology. Unfortunately, many writers investigating aspects of mutism were unaware of, or unable to apply, the basic principles of applied research, such as manipulation of an independent variable, use of a research design, and formal reliability measures. In some respects, behavior therapists using case study methodology, like their psychodynamic colleagues, claimed that various techniques were indispensable to success when this was not really supported by the data.

Behavior therapists have intervened with the selectively mute child in the clinic (Reed, 1963; Reid, Hawkins, Keutzer, McNeal, Phelps, Reid, & Mees, 1967), school (Adkins, 1975; Bauermeister & Jemail, 1975; Bednar, 1974; Brison, 1966; Colligan, Colligan, & Dilliard, 1977; Conrad, Delk, & Williams, 1974; Dmitriev & Hawkins, 1973; Rasbury, 1974; Rosenbaum & Kellman, 1973; Semenoff, Park, & Smith, 1976), home (Sluckin & Jehu, 1969), and combined settings (Nolan & Pence, 1970).

### Clinic Settings

Reed (1963) provided a quasi-behavioral analysis of four cases of selective mutism from 2000 referrals to a child guidance clinic. After analyzing these cases, he suggested that the behavior patterns of the children did not conform to the descriptions reported by Salfield (1950) and Morris (1953; see Chapter 3), but rather could be categorized into two groups. Whereas two of the children demonstrated relaxed and unresponsive behavior and appeared immature, the other two demonstrated tenseness, overreaction to fear, and concomitant anxiety. The first group purportedly learned mutism to gain attention and evade certain activities. The second group used mutism as a fear-reducing mechanism. Some common features of these children were:

1. All children were mute, responding verbally only to a few intimates over a period of several years.

2. Neurological and medical examinations suggested no abnormal findings, and all were of normal hearing on audiometric tests.

3. They failed to establish satisfactory relationships either with adults or other children.

4. They were all from homes of the working-class socioeconomic level and free from any gross material or emotional stress.

5. There was no familial incidence of mutism or other linguistic disorder.

6. In all cases, the various school staffs reported that the children were mute on admission to school at age 5.

7. None of the children were mentally defective, but all were below average in measured intelligence (as measured on the Terman-Merrill scales).

8. Analysis of test-score patterns revealed no particular weaknesses on the verbal as opposed to the nonverbal items.

9. When the children did utter complete sentences, their vocabulary, sentence structure, and articulation appeared to be at a reasonable level of development.

10. Although all four children showed definite improvement and made reasonable adaptation to adult life, they all displayed minor "psychogenic abnormalities and a lack of social drive [pp. 102-103]."

The therapeutic procedures for these children is too generally described to indicate what specific techniques were employed. Reed (1963) noted that therapy was aimed at helping them relearn social responses. For the first pair, the attention-gaining reinforcement was weakened by building up the children's self-esteem and by reinforcing other facets of their behavior. The second pair's therapy was aimed at establishing rapport and at attempting to generalize this familiarity to other clinic situations, then to individual strangers (e.g., members of the clinic staff), and finally to groups of children and adults. Also, any verbal behaviors were reinforced, and the cooperation of home and school was actively sought to generalize verbalization.

Some of the behavioral case studies present a relatively dramatic contrast to the length of treatment characteristic of much of the psychodynamic literature. Reid et al. (1967) were able to eliminate a 6-year-old girl's mutism effectively in 1 day. The treatment program was carried out in a playroom containing only a table and chairs. The intervention was based on the assumption that the presence of strangers aroused responses incompatible with speaking (e.g., fearfulness, anxiety, withdrawal, and quiescence).

The program involved several steps. In the first step, the mother was alone with the child and fed her breakfast in small portions, with receipt of portions being dependent on the child's verbal request for food. Next, the first clinician was then able to substitute for the mother in feeding the child while maintaining the verbal behavior. Gradually, two other clinicians were added to the situation, as were other children. The three follow-up sessions held on each successive week demonstrated a maintenance of verbalizations. The child's mother reported that speech began to generalize outside the family to such situations as the

Sunday school teacher and family friends. The program was presumably extended by reprogramming the child's social environment along the lines of Straughan's (1968) adaptation of Patterson's (1965) procedures (see pp. 90–92 in this volume). This consisted of setting up natural contingencies for the reinforcement of verbal initiations and responsiveness to neighbors and peers.

Not all the behavioral interventions were as brief as that reported by Reid et al. (1967). Shaw (1971) reported a 7-month treatment of a 12-year-old girl who refused to speak. From age 8 onward, she spoke only to members of her immediate family and exclusively in Dutch, although English was commonly used at home. At age 10½, following a third referral for mutism, her parents brought her to Thistletown Hospital (Rexdale, Ontario).

At the beginning of her second year in this hospital, the child was started on a series of twice-weekly intravenous injections of amobarbital sodium (7½ gr.) and methamphetamine hydrochloride (30 mg), aimed at eliminating speech inhibitions. After 4 weeks, the amobarbital sodium was stopped, but she was continued on twice-weekly injections of methamphetamine hydrochloride (20 mg IV). Presumably, the child had an intense dislike of this, and after 3 weeks of this treatment, she whispered her first word.

Thereafter, a formal program was set up that involved specific daily criteria regarding her verbal behavior, with periodic upgradings related to these criteria. Each day's minimal speech requirements were made explicit to her, as was the condition that failure to meet daily criteria would result in the aforementioned injection on the following morning. This program was continued for 7 months. The child was not formally required to speak more than once daily, with expansions instead being confined to how, where, and to whom she spoke. She exceeded this required minimal frequency increasingly as the program continued and was often able to avoid the daily injections (i.e., eight injections used for the 1st month and only two during the last 3 months). Gradually, the child began to speak. Shaw (1971) argued that the daily renewed threat situation became a conditioned aversive stimulus, which her speech automatically terminated, resulting in both operant conditioning of speech and counteraction of the anxiety by aversion relief. On a 1-year follow-up, the child was found to be maintaining normal adjustment in home, community, and school setting. She was reported using speech appropriately in all settings, had closer relationships with other family members, and had otherwise very good academic and social adjustment.

## School Settings

Treatment of mutism in school settings has been reported by a number of writers, probably because mutism is frequently first identified as a problem behavior in that setting. A number of reports have been presented in the *Journal of School Psychology* (e.g., Brison, 1966; Colligan et al., 1977; Rosenbaum & Kellman, 1973). Brison (1966) eliminated a kindergarten child's mutism by moving him to a new class and arranging for the teacher to ignore the mute behavior and nonverbal behavior that achieved results normally achieved by talking. Once the child began talking in a whisper, this behavior was reinforced with social praise. Thereafter, normal speech was also reinforced. Follow-up 3 years later indicated that the child was not viewed as a problem.

Similarly, Rosenbaum and Kellman (1973) successfully treated a third-grade mute girl by involving school personnel in various procedures. The program consisted of three phases implemented by the teacher and speech therapist. During Phase speech with an adult in a one-to-one setting was reestablished. A shaping procedure was used in two 20-minute sessions each week in which the girl received M&Ms and praise for speaking. In Phase II, a transfer of speech to the classroom through in vivo successive approximation to the classroom environment was accomplished. The teacher and peers gradually entered the individual room in the presence of the girl's speech. Phase III involved expansion of the group by requesting the girl to invite other children from her class to the speech session. After the entire class had been invited (and with concomitant teacher approval for verbal behavior in the classroom), the girl responded aloud when asked a question in front of the entire class. The authors report that approximately 2½ months following the termination of treatment, the girl was participating fully in all aspects of her classwork.

Conrad et al. (1974) treated an 11-year-old American Indian girl who purportedly had never spoken a word in a reservation classroom during her entire 5 years of schooling. A male tribal member who worked as a paraprofessional in a psychology clinic on the reservation and a male clinical psychology graduate student conducted the sessions. The interventions consisted of stimulus-fading procedures in the house with the mother because the situation was characterized by child verbalizations. Gradually, situations were changed through successive approximations until the child responded verbally to the teacher in the classroom, but at a 1-year follow-up, the girl rarely spontaneously verbalized or initiated conversation with the teacher. Although school personnel no longer considered her verbal behavior a problem at that time, it was apparently still a problem.

Bednar (1974) successfully treated a 10-year-old Mexican-American child attending public school who purportedly had never spoken a word either in school or outside his home. The program consisted of individual sessions over a 15-month period in which the therapist shaped verbal responses through the use of contingent tangible reinforcement (i.e., a penny). Seventeen sessions were necessary for the therapist to elicit a clear, audible word, which was uttered in response to a letter-naming task. At termination of the program, the child was talking to some children and whispering to his teacher. Two years after the therapy, the child was described as verbally responsive to individuals around the school.

Adkins (1975) reported the case of a young girl who did not utter any speech for 6 months after her entry into kindergarten. During the early part of her first-grade experience, a behavior modification program was established. During an initial assessment of the problem, the school staff noted that the child was receiving attention for zero-frequency speech. Thus, the treatment plan called for a complete reversal of the staff approach; that is, social reinforcement was withheld for not speaking, and several contingencies were put into effect. In the contingency program, various questions were asked that called for a verbal response on the part of the child (e.g., children were instructed to say "I want some _____" when they came in for breakfast; if the girl did not respond, she did not receive breakfast). The program continued for approximately 2 months, at which time she began talking. Unfortunately, it is impossible to determine the actual therapeutic mechanisms responsible for change in this case.

Operant reinforcement and contingency management procedures were used by Colligan et al. (1977) to treat successfully an 11-year-old boy's 6-year history of mutism. A three-phase plan was implemented by the classroom teacher with only a minimum amount of consultation from the school psychologist. The objective of Phase I was to develop the teacher into a social reinforcer. Although this was presumably accomplished, no verbalizations were elicited from the child. In Phase II the child was taught to use a tape recorder, record speech at home, and have it played in front of the teacher. (Note: Speech in the home was occurring at a low frequency.) The child was then requested to record academic tasks at school with the teacher gradually fading into the individual session. Subsequent to this, no generalization had occurred. Next, a speech contingency similar to that enacted by Adkins (1975) was established wherein the child had to say "book" in order to obtain a desk in the classroom. This procedure was effective in eliciting speech, and the child gradually began to speak in class at a level appropriate to his peers. The final stage, Phase III, was designed to program generalization. School staff engaged the child in short verbal encounters, and by the end of the school year, normal speech was established. The 21-month follow-up indicated that the child's speech was indistinguishable from that of peers. A more extended follow-up provided by Colligan (1978) suggests generally good adjustment:

> The transition to seventh grade and the large suburban junior high school did not present an easy adjustment for Peter. He came back to visit his fifth grade teacher on two occasions. On one he indicated that he had been suspended from school for smoking cigarettes in the gym with a friend. Teachers indicated that his class work was average to low-average, but of greatest significance was his regression to excessive quietness in the classroom. In part, this was believed to be a product of the tendency of the junior high school teachers to engage in more rapid-paced classroom interactions. Peter would respond verbally in the classroom if waiting time for responding was provided by the teacher. During Grade Eight he visited his fifth grade teacher once. Teacher indicates that he was almost unable to recognize him because Peter had allowed his hair to grow very long and had also grown a surprisingly substantial beard for an adolescent of this age. He had also entered the

growth spurt and was at that time approximately five feet nine inches in height. He was smiling and seemed relatively happy with himself, indicating that his grades had improved. He reported that he was receiving average grades in general, but in his favorite subject (Speech) he was earning grades of A and B (pp. 1-2).

In another school setting, Dmitriev and Hawkins (1973) successfully treated a mute girl who had remained silent despite concentrated interventions by parents, teachers, and various professionals to establish speech. The intervention consisted of eliminating social reinforcement for silence and providing specific cues for verbalizations. Results reported in Fig. 5.1 suggest that after 5 days, the child began to respond verbally to teachers' cues. Figure 5.1 suggests that an increased rate of verbalizations occurred with fewer cues. On the 22nd day of the interven-

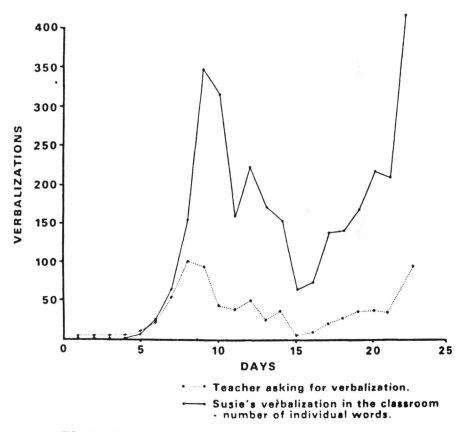

• ······• **Teacher asking for verbalization.**

   ——— **Susie's verbalization in the classroom**
   **- number of individual words.**

FIG. 5.1. The number of verbalizations in response to teacher cues in a 9-year-old mute child over 22 days. (Source: Dmitriev, V., & Hawkins, J. Susie never used to say a word. *Teaching Exceptional Children*, 1973, *6*, 68-76. Reproduced by permission.)

tion, the child spoke 421 words, or an average of 4 words for each verbal response cue from the teacher. The authors reported generalized speech and maintenance over a 4-year period. Purportedly, normal academic and social adjustment were also achieved.

Also operating in a school setting, Bauermeister and Jemail (1975) used operant procedures to treat an 8-year-old Puerto Rican child who refused to participate in classroom activities requiring verbal behaviors. Presumably, the boy communicated freely and without difficulty outside the classroom setting. Four target behaviors selected for treatment in the classroom consisted of hand raising, answering teacher questions (across homeroom and English teachers), reading aloud, and completing classroom assignments. The program was divided into four phases and was implemented by the child's homeroom and English teachers. Phase I constituted the baseline phase. The teachers were asked to continue to interact with the child in the same manner as they always had. Thus, no specific or systematic reinforcement contingency was in effect during this phase. During Phase II, both teachers were instructed to encourage the child to participate actively in class and to reinforce with praise the occurrence of the target behaviors of any "reasonable approximations." In Phase III, the homeroom teacher was explicitly asked to set goals for each class period and to praise each target behavior on each occurrence. During this time, the child also received a star from the teacher and mother, with a bicycle promised when three stars were earned. The English teacher continued the Phase III contingencies. In Phase IV, the English teacher praised the child each time a target behavior occurred, and a star was distributed at the termination of the class period. The homeroom teacher maintained the reinforcing procedures of Phase III during Phase IV class periods.

Results are reported in Table 5.1. Answering questions improved from 18.25% during baseline to 100% during the final phase; reading aloud went from 0% to 100% during baseline and the final treatment phase, respectively. The authors also reported a grade improvement that resulted in promotion to fourth grade. The 1-year follow-up suggested maintenance of the treatment gains.

TABLE 5.1
Summary of the Mean Frequency or Percentage of Target Behavior
During the Treatment Phases[a]

|                                        |        | Phase  |      |        |
| -------------------------------------- | ------ | ------ | ---- | ------ |
| Target Behavior                        | I      | II     | III  | IV     |
| Raising hand (homeroom teacher)        | 0      | 0.17   | 4    | 2.4    |
| Raising hand (English teacher)         | 0      | 0.84   | 1    | 3.8    |
| Answering question (homeroom teacher)  | 18.25% | 53.93% | 100% | 100%   |
| Reading aloud (homeroom teacher)       | 0%     | 83.33% | 100% | 100%   |
| Work completion (homeroom teacher)     | 0%     | 8%     | 56%  | 71.42% |

[a]Source: Bauermeister and Jemail (1975).

Noteworthy in this report were the focus on specific academic work and the procedure that was implemented by teachers in the classroom that only minimally interfered with regular classroom activities.

Semenoff et al. (1976) presented the case of a 4-year-old boy who had spoken normally but who, at the age of 3½, suddenly stopped talking for no apparent reason. At the time he entered a preschool, he talked only to his mother, father, maternal grandmother, and one neighborhood child. The child had some brief verbal contacts with an ice-cream man but talked to no one else throughout his preschool year. When the child entered kindergarten, he still had not talked with anyone except the same four or five people.

The intervention program extended over kindergarten, first grade, and second grade. The "speech therapy" sessions began with establishing rapport and eliciting nonverbal responses, imitation of actions and sounds, reproducing sounds on his own, speaking words alone, speaking to his teacher alone in class, and finally speaking aloud in a wider variety of situations. Although he made progress, he was still talking very little outside the speech room.

Unfortunately, when the child entered first grade the following fall, there had been a notable regression during the summer that resulted in further select speech. The initial intervention in the first grade again consisted of building trust and rapport. Thereafter, a series of nine steps were implemented that consisted of eliciting nonverbal responses, verbal mumbles, speaking in whispers, speaking before other adults, speaking before other children, speaking before a small group during regular class time, responding before the whole class, and speaking spontaneously before the whole class. The child presumably improved during the subsequent summer, and no regression occurred during the first part of the school year of the second grade. The authors noted that from January to April, the boy was responding to 100% of the questions directed to him. Moreover, the frequency of his spontaneous, initiating remarks was at the same level as the average for the second-grade classroom. Figure 5.2 shows the frequency of his spontaneous remarks compared with those of a "child taken at random." The authors counted the child's spontaneous comments during a 15-minute period of informal, seated activity when the students were allowed quiet talking. Although the data are quite limited from a scientific perspective (cf. Krumboltz & Thoresen, 1976), they could be construed as a social validity measure on outcome (see Kazdin, 1977c, and a discussion in Chapter 6 for more details). Although the authors reported no formal data, they did indicate that the child was speaking more normally in a variety of settings and to different people.

## Other Settings

Although many mute children are identified in school or clinic settings, this has not always been the primary intervention setting. Some authors employing behavioral procedures intervened across several different situations. Sluckin and Jehu (1969) report the case of a 4-year, 11-month-old girl who was first referred

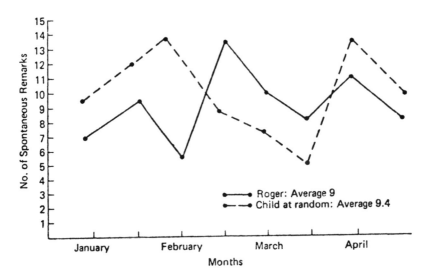

FIG. 5.2.   Spontaneous speech observed during 15-minute observations in the classroom. During each observation, a different classmate was selectied at random to be observed, and his or her spontaneous remarks were counted. The broken line on the chart shows the composite observations made for the "child at random" in the classroom. (Source: Semenoff, B., Park, C., & Smith, E. Behavioral interventions with a six-year-old elective mute. In J. D. Krumboltz & C. E. Thoresen (Eds.), *Counseling Methods*. New York: Holt, Rinehart & Winston, 1976. Reproduced by permission.)

to a child clinic because of her restricted speech in certain situations. The child was not seen at the clinic, because she was extremely fearful of strangers. In the treatment program, a psychiatric social worker first consulted with the mother on the development of the intervention plan. The child was seen in the home by the social worker, where a systematic shaping procedure with tangible reinforcement was employed. Gradually, the mother was faded out of the home while talking was reinforced. Thereafter, the child eventually began to speak to adults and children.

Nolan and Pence (1970) successfully treated a 10-year-old girl in the natural environment. The only adults she really talked to were her parents, but she had also whispered to a female neighbor and to a few select children. Over an 8-month period, the child was involved in a series of interventions, some of which occurred simultaneously. In the first attempt to manipulate the girl's verbal behavior, the mother was instructed to inform the child that all nonvocal behavior could no longer occur in the car. The mother enforced this contingency by ignoring nonverbal communication while going to and from school. After 3 days of this contingency, the child began to whisper. The mother was next directed to turn up the volume on the radio a little louder each day. Using this fading procedure, the child, on occasions, emitted normal speech. Thereafter, a variety of management programs were implemented across many situations and individuals. For example, a teacher employed a token economy and rewarded all verbal behaviors in the school. Gradually, the child spoke in a normal fashion, and the authors reported normal speech upon a 1-year follow-up. A 5-year postcontact suggested that the client was an active high school student in a regular public school system with no unusual problems (Nolan, 1978).

Rasbury, (1974) described an in vivo desensitization program designed to reinstate normal verbal communication in an 11-year-old girl who was selectively mute for approximately 6 years. The mutism had developed shortly after an aversive incident (unspecified) that occurred on a school bus. Eight months prior to the desensitization program, the child was first invoved in traditional play therapy (cf. Axline, 1947) and then in behavior therapy emphasizing positive reinforcement for language imitation (e.g., Lovaas, Berberich, Perloff, & Schaeffer, 1966). Neither of these programs successfully reinstated the child's verbal behavior. A desensitization program was therefore implemented in the family car on the way to school, because it was observed that speech became increasingly inhibited, the closer the child came to the school setting. Each school morning, the child was required to read aloud a set of sentences printed on index cards. The sentences described various activities that the child could become involved in at school, such as recess, art, and so forth. Successful reading of each card allowed her to attend the activity that day. Movement up a hierarchy was based on speaking in a normal tone of voice (defined subjectively by the father) and speaking for 3 successive days. Movement up the hierarchy was based on speaking in the presence of the father in close proximity to the school and other people, and finally on speaking to individuals outside the family without the father present. The complete program involved 140 sessions (1 per day), each of 10 minutes duration, with 15 steps in the hierarchy. Although the program was successful, the child met an untimely death a year later.

Norman and Broman (1970) treated a 12-year-old mute boy who had not said a word in more than 8 years outside his immediate home through positive reinforcement procedures. Visual feedback from a volume-level meter was employed to induce sounds and raise speech volume. Reinforcement (e.g., a soft drink) was also used to increase rate of speech and to generalize it to other situations. The sound meter contained a background divided into red (loudest sounds) and black (low- or no-sound regions). The intervention lasted for 44 sessions and from 40 to 400 trials per session (range: 30-60 minutes per session). The target variables consisted of three measures: The child's voice either moved the meter needle into a black or red region, or no response was made. Results reported in Fig. 5.3 show that the program increased responses in the red and decreased the percentage of no responses. Black-region responses also gradually decreased over sessions. During the last session, the child responded to 80% of the questions from one adult and 54% from a new person. At an 18-month follow-up, the child was still speaking. The authors reported that school personnel trained in behavior modification procedures took over the school treatment program.

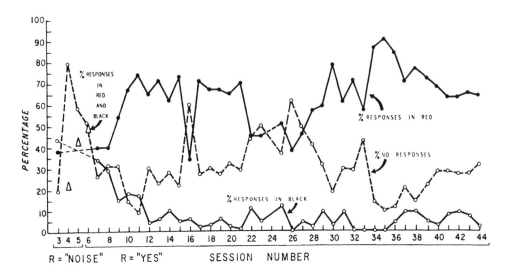

FIG. 5.3.   A record of subject's responses to HB with no one else in the room. Note the "all-or-none" pattern of responding in most sessions; subject either gave a reinforced response (red) or did not respond. In Sessions 4, 5, and 6, responses in "red" and "black" were accidently combined during recording the data and are represented by triangles. (Source: Norman, A., & Broman, H. J. Volume feedback and generalization techniques in shaping speech of an electively mute boy: A case study. *Perceptual and Motor Skills,* 1970, *31,* 463–470. Reprinted by permission of authors and publisher.)

## FORMAL SINGLE-CASE DESIGNS

In some of the selective mutism research, authors reported more formalized designs to evaluate their treatment programs. As noted earlier in the chapter, the distinction between the reports presented in this section and those already discussed in the case study section is somewhat arbitrary. Again, the behavioral literature is reviewed by setting.

### Clinic and Combined Settings

In a booth designed especially for treatment of autistic and selectively mute children, Blake and Moss (1967) assessed a 4-year-old girl who had no communicative speech or imitative skills.[1] Baseline assessment revealed a high fre-

---

[1]The child in the Blake and Moss (1967) report does not qualify as a selective mute child by criteria discussed in Chapter 1. Although their definition of elective mutism is quite different from that of the majority of writers in this area, the procedure is described here because of its potential usefulness in the treatment of selective mutism.

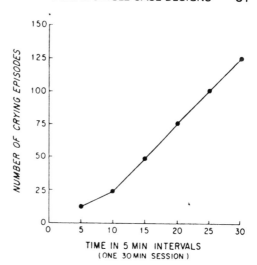

FIG. 5.4. Baseline assessment: Number of crying episodes (duration of 5 sec. or more). (Source: Blake, P., & Moss, T. The development of socialization skills in an electively mute child. *Behavior Research & Therapy,* 1967, *5,* 349-356. Reproduced by permission.)

quency of crying episodes (see Fig. 5.4). To elicit sounds from the child, an instrument called a "color organ" was used as a positive reinforcer. The instrument (described by Fineman, 1966) translates sounds uttered into a microphone into an array of fusing colors on a screen. Intensities of the colors vary in proportion to the intensities of sounds emitted into the microphone. After baseline, in 40 half-hour sessions, the child was taught to make eye contact with the therapist and to obey instructions. The operant crying was also extinguished (see Fig. 5.5). During the intervention, the child learned nonverbal imitative behavior, such as hand clapping and ear pulling, and verbal imitative behavior, such as saying "hi" (see Fig. 5.6). Beginning with Session 12, verbal responses were attempted. This was begun with a free operant training procedure in which every descrete sound (with a 2-second interval between sounds) was rewarded

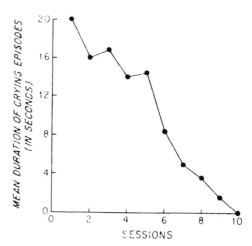

FIG. 5.5. Extinction of operant crying. (Source: Blake, P., & Moss, T. The development of socialization skills in an electively mute child. *Behavior Research & Therapy,* 1967, *5,* 349-356. Reproduced by permission.)

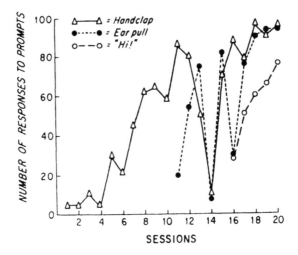

FIG. 5.6.   Imitative responses over 20 sessions. (Source: Blake, P., & Moss, T.
The development of socialization skills in an electively mute child. *Behavior
Research & Therapy*, 1967, *5*, 349-356. Reproduced by permission.)

with a food reinforcer. The child's vocal output increased dramatically (see Fig.
5.7). Starting with Session 21, differential reinforcement was begun for approximations of the word *eat*. A discrimination between the sounds *hi* and *ee* was
also successfully established (see Fig. 5.8). During Session 21 and thereafter,
play periods were begun (e.g., singing sounds) in which some verbal behavior
was generalized beyond the booth. Although the program was labeled a success,
the sounds *hi* and *ee* were the only discriminable responses in the subject's
repertoire upon completion of the program. According to a later report (Moss &

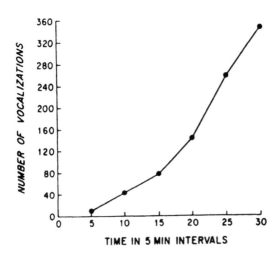

FIG. 5.7.   Number of vocalizations
(free operant) with reinforcements:
Session 12. (Source: Blake, P., &
Moss, T. The development of socialization skills in an electively mute
child. *Behavior Research & Therapy*,
1967, *5*, 349-356. Reproduced by
permission.)

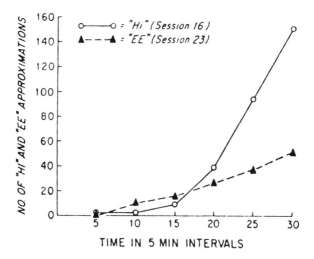

FIG. 5.8.   Differential reinforcement of verbal response approximations. (Source: Blake, P., & Moss, T. The development of socialization skills in an electively mute child. *Behavior Research & Therapy,* 1967, *5,* 349-356. Reproduced by permission.)

Blake, 1970), this was due to the parents' marital difficulties, which prompted them to remove the child from therapy before any realistic measure of the success of the treatment could be obtained. However, in the Moss and Blake (1970) report, the authors describe the continuation of the treatment program for the child.

In the report, the authors note that the girl had not progressed beyond learning to say "dye-dye" (for bye-bye) and had maintained her learning of "hi" as a greeting, with a wave of her hand. The new intervention strategy, introduced after an 8-month lapse, consisted of the use of operant training by one therapist combined with psychodynamic therapy by another therapist, who facilitated the verbal and social development of the child. Specifically, the first therapist worked with the child in the teaching booth, using the conditioning procedures used in the Blake and Moss (1967) report. In addition to these *formal* speech training sessions, the second therapist conducted "social sessions" where no reinforcements were used other than social ones (e.g., smiles, caresses, approval). The purpose of these social sessions was to generalize the new responses. In addition, the second therapist, in cooperation with the child's mother, worked to establish toilet training, dressing and undressing by the girl without help, and the management of eating utensils other than a spoon.

The authors report that during the subsequent 3 months, further progress was made, particularly in the development of such social skills as toilet training and learning to dress and undress herself. Unfortunately, although the girl demonstrated the ability to speak several words clearly, and sometimes spontaneously, she proved extremely resistant to any real or lasting development of verbal skills. Thereafter, it was decided to place her in hospitalized day care. But again, her parents withdrew her from treatment. The authors imply that behavior therapy and psychodynamic therapy worked well together, but because the case was generally unsuccessful, it cannot be verified.

Wulbert, Nyman, Snow, and Owen (1973) compared stimulus-fading techniques to contingency management in the treatment of a 6-year-old selectively mute girl. Purportedly, the child had not spoken in kindergarten, in years of Sunday school, or in 1 year of preschool. The treatment procedures, in part, were similar to those employed by Reid et al. (1967) in that the child's mother rewarded the child for verbal and motor responses to scheduled tasks while a stranger slowly entered the room and then gradually administered the task items as the mother left the room. A time-out contingency for nonresponse to task

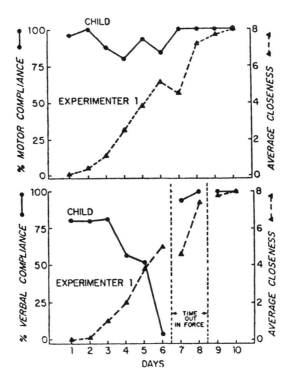

FIG. 5.9. Percent of compliance to demands for verbal and motor response during experimental periods as Experimenter 1 faded in to stimulus control. A time-out contingency was in effect on Days 7 and 8. (Source: Wulbert, M., Nyman, B. A., Snow, I., & Owen, Y. The efficacy of stimulus fading and contingency management in the treatment of elective mutism: A case study. *Journal of Applied Behavior Analysis*, 1973, 6, 435–441. Copyright by Society for the Experimental Analysis of Behavior, Inc., reproduced by permission.)

items was also employed. Control periods consisted of a stranger administering the same tasks to the child under the same contingencies but without the presence of the mother or the use of stimulus fading. Experimental and control periods were alternated during each treatment session. Figure 5.9 shows the course of the fading process for Experimenter 1. During the first 6 days of treatment, as Experimenter 1 moved closer to the child, her motor behavior dropped off slightly from what it had been when Experimenter 1 was not present. As Experi-

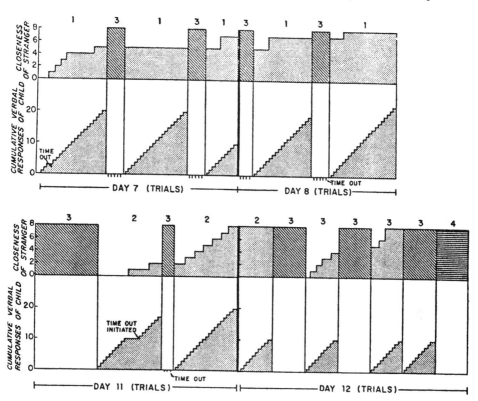

FIG. 5.10. Cumulative verbal response of the child during experimental and control periods. Experimenters are numberd in the order in which they were faded in to stimulus control. Numbers at the top of the graph refer to experimenters. Days 7 and 8: Experimenter 1 administered the experimental periods; Experimenter 3, the control periods. Day 11: Experimenter 2 faded in to stimulus control, and Experimenter 3 administered the control periods. Day 12: Experimenter 3 continued to administer the control periods until he was completely faded in to stimulus control. Experimenter 4 then administered the control period. (Source: Wulbert, M., Nyman, B. A., Snow, I., & Owen, Y. The efficacy of stimulus fading and contingency management in the treatment of elective mutism: A case study. *Journal of Applied Behavior Analysis*, 1973, *6*, 435–441. Copyright by Society for the Experimental Analysis of Behavior, Inc., reproduced by permission.)

menter 1 moved closer, the child's verbal behavior dropped off completely. The child made neither verbal nor motor responses to Experimenter 3 during the control periods. On Day 7, when the time-out contingency was put into effect, a failure to respond resulted in the child being placed in a darkened room for 1 minute. With the time-out contingency in effect, the child responded to all verbal and motor task items presented during experimental sessions. The child responded to 100% of all cues for verbal and motor behavior on Days 8, 9, and 10, as Experimenter 1 moved closer and acquired complete stimulus control.

The time-out contingency had a very different effect in the control sessions than it did in the experimental sessions. Figure 5.10 shows the cumulative verbal responses of the child during experimental and control periods. Figure 5.11 shows the number of trials required to fade in successive experimenters. Whereas the time-out contingency for nonresponse was found to facilitate the treatment if combined with stimulus fading, it was completely ineffective without stimulus fading. Figure 5.11 shows there was a definite trend indicating that each successive experimenter was adapted to more quickly by the child. The program was successfully moved to the school, with Experimenter 7 (the child's teacher) obtaining a response from the child. Although the study offers evidence that the treatment of selective mutism is affected through the combined use of a stimulus-fading procedure and contingency management, there was no evidence that full verbalization (normal) was achieved in the school.

Van der Kooy and Webster (1975) used a variety of behavioral procedures to treat a 6-year-old child who had not spoken in most social situations outside the

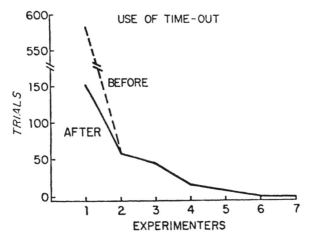

FIG. 5.11.   Number of trials to fade in successive experimenters to stimulus control. (Source: Wulbert, M., Nyman, B. A., Snow, I., & Owen, Y. The efficacy of stimulus fading and contingency management in the treatment of elective mutism: A case study. *Journal of Applied Behavior Analysis*, 1973, *6*, 435–441. Copyright by Society for the Experimental Analysis of Behavior, Inc., reproduced by permission.)

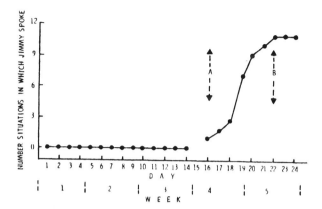

FIG. 5.12.  Jimmy's speech in different social situations at camp. See text for a description of the selective mutism situations. He was absent on Day 15. *A* indicates the point at which the treatment program started. *B* indicates the point at which extra staff attention was faded out. (Source: Van der Kooy, D., & Webster, C. D. A rapidly effective behavior modification program for an electively mute child. *Journal of Behavior Therapy and Experimental Psychiatry*, 1975, *6*, 149–152. Reproduced by permission.)

home, including school, for approximately 2 years. The program was conducted in a summer camp and involved components of avoidance conditioning, positive social reinforcement, generalization procedures, and the fading of extra attention. An initial intervention procedure consisted of dunking the child in a swimming pool, a procedure that has ethical implications (see a discussion of ethical issues in Chapter 7). A program was instituted to generalize the child's speech outside the swimming pool. Figure 5.12 shows that the summer-camp day was arbitrarily divided so as to show a record of the boy's progress in generalization. Eleven social-situation categories were listed: verbal greeting to staff or peer in the morning; speech to peers in free-play sessions in the morning; speech on a trip to the pool; speech to one person in the pool; speech in the showers; speech in the change room; speech at lunch; speech during the afternoon; and verbal good-bye to a staff member or peer at night.

Similar to Straughan's (1968) findings, the authors observed that the fading program was greatly assisted by peers who reinforced the child by verbally responding to him and by complying to his verbal requests. Although likely a useful therapeutic procedure, this did not appear to be a planned part of the program. A 6-month follow-up indicated that the child was speaking appropriately in the school, demonstrating both durability and generalization of the program.

Some authors have treated mutism along with other major behavioral disturbances. Munford, Reardon, Liberman, and Allen (1976) reported successful treatment of a 17-year-old girl, diagnosed "hysterical neurosis," who demonstrated incessant coughing at the rate of 40 to 50 coughs per minute over a 4-year period and selective mutism for 2 of the last 4 years. The primary intervention procedure for the mutism involved shaping speech using home visits requested by the child as the reinforcer. The shaping procedure included several major components: First, muscles requiring control over shoulder, head, and neck areas were shaped. To reduce rigidity in these areas, the girl was instructed to perform progressively ordered exercises that resulted in accomplishing neck rolls, tongue extensions, parting teeth, and so forth. A major goal was to increase the girl's control over inhalation and exhalation, which in turn led to the objective of sound producing beginning with closures, and then moving to consonant and vowel combinations. The final cluster of behavior focused on the pronunciation of words, followed by phrases and sentences.

An early version of the changing-criterion design (see Chapter 6) with a treatment reversal was used to assess the effects of instructions, feedback, and the home reinforcement contingency. As Fig. 5.13 suggests, the shaping procedure was slow, with the program extending over 24 weeks. Within 6 weeks following treatment, the girl was discharged from the hospital demonstrating appropriate and fluent speech. The authors suggest that at this point, the cough frequency and volume were reduced by about half of the former baseline rate. Presumably, the lessened frequency was attributable to the resumption of speech, which was incompatible with coughing.

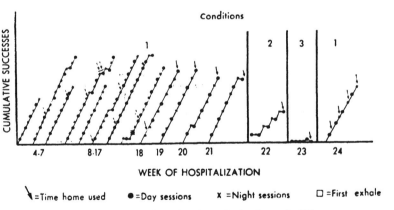

FIG. 5.13.   Successes in meetings changing criteria of speech skills program. (Condition 1: Criteria specified, feedback given, contingent reinforcement of time home: Condition 2: Criteria specified, no feedback given, noncontingent reinforcement: Condition 3: No criteria specified, no feedback, noncontingent reinforcement. Weeks 4–7—neck, mouth movement; 8–17—lip control, breathing; 18—sounds, words; 20—phrases/volume; 21–24—sentences and rate.) (Source: Munford, P. R., Reardon, D., Liberman, R. P., & Allen, L. Behavioral treatment of hysterical coughing and mutism: A case study. *Journal of Consulting and Clinical Psychology*, 1976, *44*, 1008–1014. Copyright (1976) by the American Psychological Association. Reprinted by permission.)

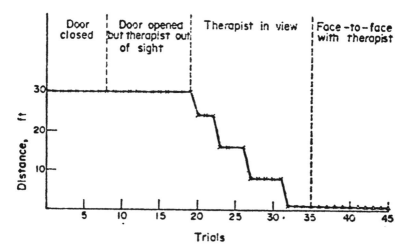

FIG. 5.14. Stages of desensitization: X-verbal responses to the written word; ▲-verbal responses to the spoken word on tape; △-verbal responses to the therapist. (Source: Scott, E. A desensitization programme for the treatment of mutism in a seven-year-old girl: A case report. *Journal of Child Psychology and Psychiatry*, 1977, *18*, 263–270. Reprinted by permission.)

Although the elimination of mutism can be partly attributed to the treatment program, concurrent individual, family, and ancillary therapies make interpretation difficult (cf. Kratochwill et al., 1979). For example, throughout the client's hospitalization, daily individual therapy sessions were held to maintain motivation to continue therapy. The girl was also socially reinforced for her daily achievements. Finally, weekly family therapy sessions were held to provide a common forum for each member's reaction to the hospitalization and to promote generalization of the program. It was noted that the child was symptom free 41 months following discharge. She also completed two quarters of college with excellent grades. Munford (1978) noted that the client continues to speak appropriately and fluently and remains symptom free.

Some writers have combined desensitization and operant methods of behavior therapy to treat selective mutism. Scott (1977) reports the case of a 6-year, 5-month-old girl who had never spoken outside of her immediate family. Therapy was instituted consequent on the consideration that the child had established a good relationship with the therapist during previous psychotherapeutic sessions. The program involved gradually introducing the therapist into the hospital treatment room while the child read into a tape recorder. The child was presented with a picture under which were listed 10 simple questions. On presentation of the task, she switched on the recorder, read the questions, and then answered in a sentence. Rewards were also provided. The child sought close physical contact with the therapist, so while listening to the playback, she was allowed to sit on the therapist's knee. At the end of the entire session, she was also rewarded with a packet of sweets.

Figure 5.14 shows the results of the desenitization procedure wherein increases in interaction with the therapist are presented. The program involved gradually introducing the therapist into the treatment room while the child read into a tape recorder. Thereafter, the child's verbal response to the written word were transferred to the spoken word by degrees. Finally, the classroom teacher helped transfer the activities to the classroom, where six children were included in the program. This intervention program took place over a period of 4 weeks. Although the plan appeared effective, no follow-up results were reported. The behavior change was effectively generalized.

## School Settings

Straughan and his associates (Straughan, 1968; Straughan, Potter, & Hamilton, 1965) documented several cases of successful interventions with children experiencing speech and language problems. Although some of these involved work with "delayed speech" or "schizophrenic mutism" (Straughan, 1968), the same procedures were used to treat selective mutism. In a report designed to extend the application of a procedure originally used for modifying hyperactive behavior (see Patterson, 1965), Straughan et al. (1965) employed a reinforcement technique consisting of a flashing light that signaled that a reward (e.g., candy, points) toward a party had been earned to treat a 14-year-old mute boy in a school for the mentally retarded. Characteristics of the youth included: (1) remaining silent except with intimate friends; (2) showing unusual timidity and shyness; (3) no known neurological deficiencies; (4) reported mute from his entrance in school at age 6; (5) doing unsatisfactory academic work; and (6) scoring in the deficient range on intelligence tests.

The treatment program was divided into four phases: (1) preliminary observation $(A_1)$; (2) systematic observation $(A_2)$; (3) treatment $(B_1)$; and (4) posttreatment observation $(B_2)$. In $A_2$, the youth's behavior was carefully recorded for 21 days, 20 minutes per day. Variables recorded during this experiment included looking at another person, smiling, motor responses, no responses, and talking. Results reported in Fig. 5.15 indicated that the teacher's questions to the youth varied from a low of 1 question on Day 19 to a high of 143 questions during the observation period on Day 44. Even after 15 days of treatment, there were still some days when the youth did not respond during the few minutes of the observation period. A further breakdown of the data is reported in Table 5.2. The results suggest that the frequency of talking, talking in response to the teacher, and peer vocal responses to the youth were higher during treatment and after treatment phases. The data offer support for the hypothesis that Patterson's (1965) technique for manipulating classroom behavior was effective in changing the selective mutism. A 1-year follow-up documented that the youth was still talking

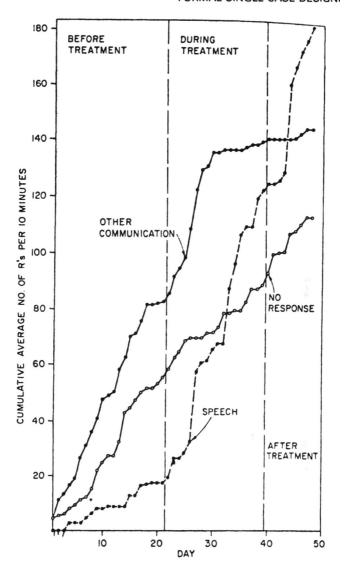

FIG. 5.15.  Daily cumulative average response frequencies to the teacher per 10-minute observation period. "Other communication" consisted of smiling or looking at the teacher or making an appropriate motor response. (Source: Straughan, J. H. The application of operant conditioning to the treatment of elective mutism. In H. Sloane & B. MacAuly (Eds.), *Operant procedures in remedial speech and language training.* Boston: Houghton Mifflin & Co., 1968. Reproduced by permission.)

TABLE 5.2
The Total Frequency of Talking, Talking in Response to Instructor,
and Peer Vocal Approaches to Gene[a]

|  | Total Observation Time | Frequency of Talking | Frequency per 10 Minutes |
|---|---|---|---|
| Before treatment | 420 min | 97 | 2.31 |
| During treatment | 180 min | 493 | 27.39 |
| After treatment | 270 min | 852 | 31.56 |

$\chi^2 = 1008.16$; $P < 0.001$; $df = 2$.

Talking in Response to Instructor

|  | No. of Instructor's Questions | No. of Vocal Responses | Proportion of Vocal Responses |
|---|---|---|---|
| Before treatment | 311 | 35 | 0.11 |
| During treatment | 195 | 105 | 0.54 |
| After treatment | 292 | 178 | 0.61 |

$\chi^2 = 106.62$; $P < 0.001$; $df = 2$.

Peer Vocal Approaches to Gene

|  | Length of Observation Time | Number of Approaches | Number per per 10 Minutes |
|---|---|---|---|
| Before treatment | 420 min | 15 | 0.36 |
| During treatment | 180 min | 28 | 1.56 |
| After treatment | 270 min | 139 | 5.15 |

$\chi^2 = 183.93$; $P < 0.001$; $df = 2$.
[a]Source: Straughan, Potter, & Hamilton, 1965.

although his responsiveness was not as high as was observed immediately follow-ing the program. Straughan et al. (1965) suggested that peer reactions play an important role in maintaining the reinforced behavior after the experimental program is terminated.

Some authors labeled children experiencing a low frequency of verbalizations across situations electively mute. In the only report in which a group of school children ($N = 8$) were involved in a program to modify low-frequency verbaliza-tion, Calhoun and Koenig (1973) documented a successful treatment consisting of rewards contingent on classroom verbal interaction. The group was equally divided, with four children serving as the nontreated controls and four receiving the treatment suited to each individual child's problem and level of social skills. Results reported in Fig. 5.16 suggest that a change in verbal behavior occurred from approximately 17 words per 30 minutes of observation to approximately 60 per minute for the treated group. Although a 1-year follow-up suggested continued relatively high rates of verbalization, no data were reported on the generalizability of talking.

Williamson and his associates (Williamson, Sanders, Sewell, Haney, & White, 1977a; Williamson, Sewell, Sanders, Haney, & White, 1977b) reported the successful treatment of elective mutism and "reluctant" speech. The first case Williamson et al. (1977b) treated was one mute child using shaping with modeling, escape and reinforcement, and shaping and fading. In the second case, shaping with modeling, reinforcement and reinforcer sampling with stimulus fading, and reinforcement and reinforcement fading were employed. Results for Case 1 and Case 2 are reported in Figs. 5.17 and 5.18, respectively. The frequency of speaking in certain environments (e.g., school) increased for both cases. Follow-up data gathered from 1 month to 1 year, later documented that the changes were maintained or improved.

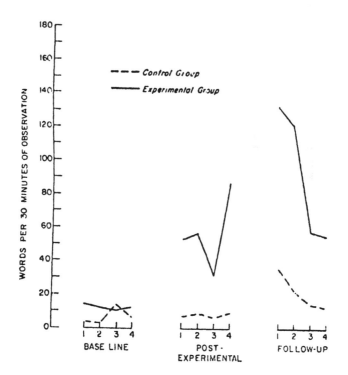

FIG. 5.16.  Changes in verbal behavior as a function of treatments and time. (Source: Calhoun, J., & Koenig, K. P. Classroom modification of elective mutism. *Behavior Therapy*, 1973, *4*, 700–702. Reproduced by permission.)

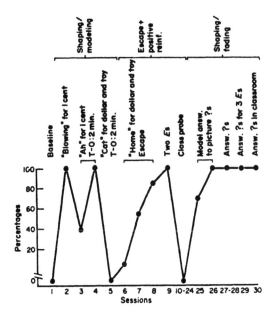

FIG. 5.17. The percentage of prompted verbal responses for shaping modeling, escape and positive reinforcement, and shaping fading phases. (Source: Williamson, D. A., Sanders, S. H., Sewell, W. R., Haney, J. N., & White, D. The behavioral treatment of elective mutism: Two case studies. *Journal of Behavior Therapy & Experimental Psychiatry*, 1977, 8, 143–149. (a) Reproduced by permission.)

In a second report, two cases of "reluctant speech" were successfully treated using contingency management procedures in the school, home, and clinic. In the first case, a token economy program was implemented in which a 45-minute class party was made contingent upon the child making 45 verbalizations to other children during recess. Each instance of speaking was immediately rewarded with a token. After recess, the boy traded the tokens for stars that were placed on a chart. His verbal behavior during recess was recorded by a behavioral technician, and the reinforcement procedures were administered by the teacher. Results of the token procedure are reported in Fig. 5.19. After the boy had earned the class party on the 5th day of treatment, the reinforcer was changed to privileges (e.g., being first in the lunch line). Two 30-minute follow-up observations 1 year later suggested that the changes were maintained, and the boy was one of the most popular children in the class.

In the second case, the baseline and treatment procedures were implemented in the clinic and home. The procedures in the clinic were conducted in an isolated room with a one-way mirror so that the mother could learn appropriate behavioral interaction patterns via modeling by the therapist. Figures 5.20 and 5.21 show the results of the baseline observations and treatment procedures for both prompted and spontaneous speech. The treatment consisted of a contingency management token economy program in which the boy received tokens contingent upon either prompted or spontaneous speech. Follow-up data collected 2 months after treatment suggested that prompted speech remained near 90% and that spontaneous speech had increased considerably.

A similar contingency management procedure was implemented in the child's home environment during the regular treatment period. This program consisted of token reinforcement of spontaneous comments made by the boy to persons outside his immediate family. Tokens earned in this setting (as they were in the clinic) were exchanged for toys, privileges, and so forth. Figure 5.22 shows that the spontaneous verbalizations to nonfamily persons increased from a frequency of zero per week during baseline to 56 per week at the end of treatment. Two-month and 1-month follow-ups documented maintenance of the therapeutic results.

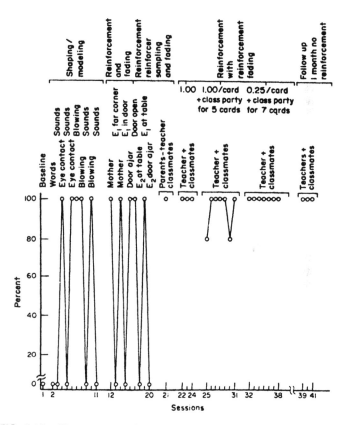

FIG. 5.18. The percentage of prompted verbal responses for Case II during shaping/modeling; reinforcement, reinforcement stimulus fading, reinforcer sampling; reinforcement/reinforcement fading; and follow-up phases. (Source: Williamson, D. A., Sanders, S. H., Sewell, W. R., Haney, J. N., & White, D. The behavior treatment of elective mutism: Two case studies. *Journal of Behavior Therapy & Experimental Psychiatry*, 1977, *8*, 143-149. (a) Reproduced by permission.)

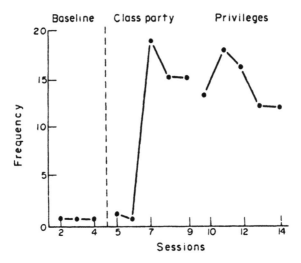

FIG. 5.19. The frequency of verbalization made by Mike (Class 1) to other classmates during recess. (Source: Williamson, D. A., Sewell, W. R., Sanders, S. H., Haney, J. N., & White, D. The treatment of reluctant speech using contingency management procedures. *Journal of Behavior Therapy & Experimental Psychiatry,* 1977, *8,* 151–156. (b) Reproduced by permission.)

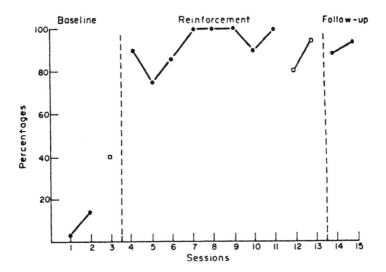

FIG. 5.20. The percentages of prompted verbal responses made by Kenneth (Case 2) to the therapist or his brother while in the clinic setting are represented by the dark circles. The open squares represent the percentages of prompted verbalizations made in the presence of a "stranger" who never delivered reinforcement. Each session lasted 15 minutes. (Source: Williamson, D. A., Sewell, W. R., Sanders, S. H., Haney, J. N., & White, D. The treatment of reluctant speech using contingency management procedures. *Journal of Behavior Therapy & Experimental Psychiatry,* 1977, *8,* 151–156. (b) Reproduced by permission.)

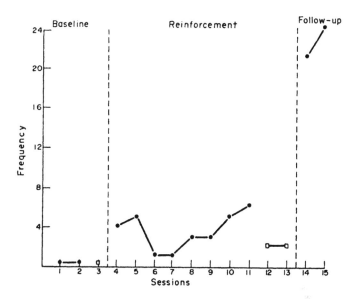

FIG. 5.21.  The frequency of spontaneous verbalizations made by Kenneth (Case 2) in the presence of the therapist and his brother (dark circles) or in the presence of a "stranger" who never reinforced his verbal behavior (open squares). Each session lasted 15 minutes. (Source: Williamson, D. A., Sewell, W. R., Sanders, S. H., Haney, J. N., & White, D. The treatment of reluctant speech using contingency management procedures. *Journal of Behavior Therapy & Experimental Psychiatry,* 1977, *8,* 151–156. (b) Reproduced by permission.)

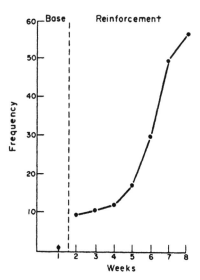

FIG. 5.22.  The frequency of spontaneous speech to nonfaculty persons made by Kenneth (Case 2), as recorded by his mother over an 8-week period. (Source: Williamson, D. A., Sewell, W. R., Sanders, S. H., Haney, J. N., & White, D. The treatment of reluctant speech using contingency management procedures. *Journal of Behavior Therapy & Experimental Psychiatry,* 1977, *8,* 151–156. (b) Reproduced by permission.)

97

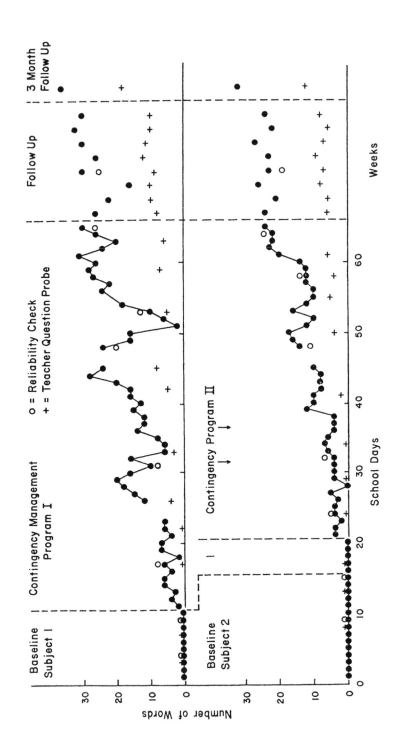

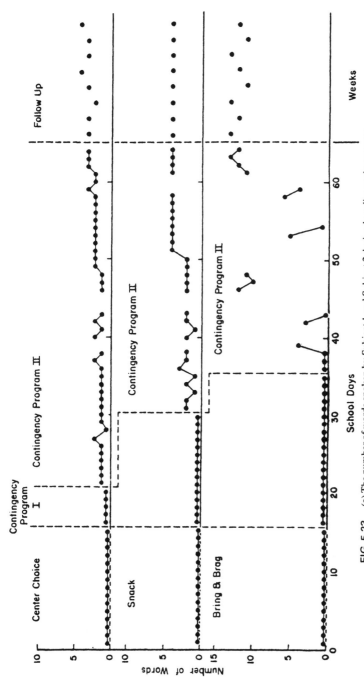

FIG. 5.23. (a) The number of words spoken by Subject 1 and Subject 2 during baseline and treatment phases across all settings where behavior was observed. Open circles represent reliability checks. Stars indicate teacher question probes in the generalization settings. Missing data for Shannon refer to those days when the subject was absent from school. Follow-up data were gathered in the classroom and generalization setting over eight weeks and upon return to school the following fall. (b) The number of words spoken by Subject 2 across three settings over baseline, treatment, and follow-up phases. Open circles represent reliability checks. Stars indicate teacher question probes in the generalization settings. Missing data reflect those days when the subject was absent from school. Follow-up data were gathered in the classroom and generalization setting over eight weeks and upon return to school the following fall.

Some authors developing programs for selective mutism applied treatments across settings within the school (Griffith, Schnelle, McNees, Bissinger, & Huff, 1975; Piersel & Kratochwill, 1981). Piersel and Kratochwill (1981) report the treatment of the selectively mute behavior of a kindergarten boy and his preschool sister by their respective classroom teachers using a contingency management program. The package, employing extinction, mild aversive procedures, and positive reinforcement, was implemented across the two subjects in a multiple baseline design. Any verbalization emitted by the children was immediately reinforced. Following the implementation of the program across the two subjects, it was necessary to target specific class activities (i.e., center choice, snacks, and bring and brag) and to implement specific contingencies sequentially for each of these selected activities to elicit and maintain speech for one of the children.

Results reported in Fig. 5.23 demonstrate an increase in verbal bahavior for both subjects during the treatment phases. On the 21st day, the aversive procedures were added to the reinforcement program for the second child. The bottom portion of Fig. 5.23 presents the results of the intervention across the three situations. The revised contingency package was effective in increasing verbalizations. Whereas the top portion of the figure represents the total frequency of words for subject 2, the bottom portion represents the number of words spoken for subject 2 during the targeted settings. The words spoken have been added to Patrick's graph to represent the total frequency of words collapsed across settings. Therefore, each setting represents words per day, and the top portion of the graph summarizes these and other verbalizations for the relative comparisons with Shannon.

Follow-up data gathered at weekly intervals until the end of the school year suggested that each subject maintained a level of verbalizations consistent with that established at the end of the formal program. A 6-month follow-up after the school year suggested that both subjects were talking to teachers and peers and were regarded as normal in social functioning.

Griffith et al. (1975) treated a 6-year-old mute boy who was enrolled in a first-grade special education class and normal first-grade reading and gym classes. After a baseline series in these three settings, a reinforcement system for peer-prompted speech and spontaneous speech was employed in the three settings in a multiple baseline fashion. In the reading class intervention, the child was given 1 point each time he spoke to a peer. He redeemed 10 points for 15 minutes of free time approximately 3 hours later in the homeroom class. In the homeroom class, the reinforcement contengencies, which had previously worked as a reading class reinforcer, had no effect as a homeroom class reinforcer and were thus changed on the 38th day to a response-cost procedure. Reinforcement contingencies identical to those in the homeroom were initiated in the same sequence in the gym class. However, the points-for-speech procedure had no effect, and the response-cost procedure was initiated on Day 48.

Results reported in Fig. 5.24 show the percent of the subject's responses to peer prompting in the three classes. Figure 5.25 shows the spontaneous speech to peers per 5-minute periods in the three classroom situations. The data reveal similar results to those reported in Fig. 5.24. (Note that the effects of the response-cost procedure coincide with those shown in the prompted speech graphs.) Approximately 3 months after·the intervention program was terminated, the child was placed in a normal second-grade classroom. Six measurements, each taken there over a 40-minute period, produced data suggesting that the treatment gains remained durable.

Nash and his associates (Nash, Thorpe, Andrews, & Davis, 1979) used a package program consisting of prompting, modeling, chaining, role playing, and reinforcement contingencies either separately or in combination to treat three cases of selective mutism. The first subject was a 5-year-old girl whose language development was normal until the age of 2, at which time she stopped speaking to anyone other than her family members. However, it was reported that she did speak with playmates. The child also refused to participate in church and nursery schools.

The second subject was a 9-year-old girl who only rarely responded to the learning disabilities classroom teacher's questioning. The girl occasionally made spontaneous statements during recess or during free time. However, her speech appeared to be selective, and she frequently refused to speak to relatives, especially males.

The third subject was an 8-year-old boy who would not speak to anyone at school but would occasionally speak to some of his classmates while playing at home. After 7 months in a classroom for emotionally distrubed children, the boy began whispering to his teacher. The authors established three treatment goals for the subjects: (1) response to teachers and other adults in individual and group settings; (2) interaction with peers; and (3) spontaneous language in everyday settings. Each subject was involved in a baseline–treatment (AB) assessment strategy. During baseline, Subject 1 made one verbal response during 8 days of Distar Language I (Engelmann, Osborn, & Engelmann, 1972) and Distar Reading I (Engelmann & Bruner, 1974) lessons. Following 3 weeks of the use of the treatment package across behaviors and settings, the child demonstrated verbal compliance from the teacher and friend in the class setting. A 2-year follow-up indicated that the girl was fully compliant to requests for both verbal and nonverbal responses.

During baseline, Subject 2 imitated the *h* sound on the 1st day, but only after it was requested 50 times. The child continued to comply on the 2nd and 3rd days but refused to say words when requested on the 4th day. In the treatment phase, the child's correct responses were reinforced with praise plus a note to her parents. Presumably, the other (or some) package components were also employed. The authors note that full compliance was achieved when other children and.another teacher and aide were included in the instructional settings. Other

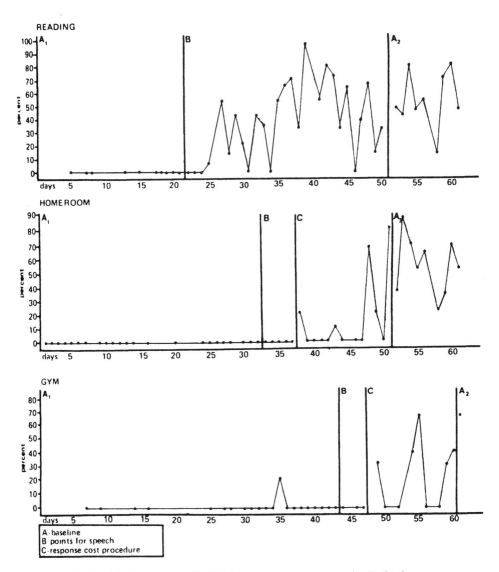

FIG. 5.24. The percent of subject's responses to peer prompting in the three classes measured: reading class, homeroom, and gym class. (Source: Griffith, E. E., Schnelle, J. R., McNees, M. P., Bissinger, C., & Huff, T. M. Elective mutism in a first grader: The remendiation of a complex behavioral problem. *Journal of Abnormal Child Psychology*, 1975, *3*, 127–134. Reproduced by permission.)

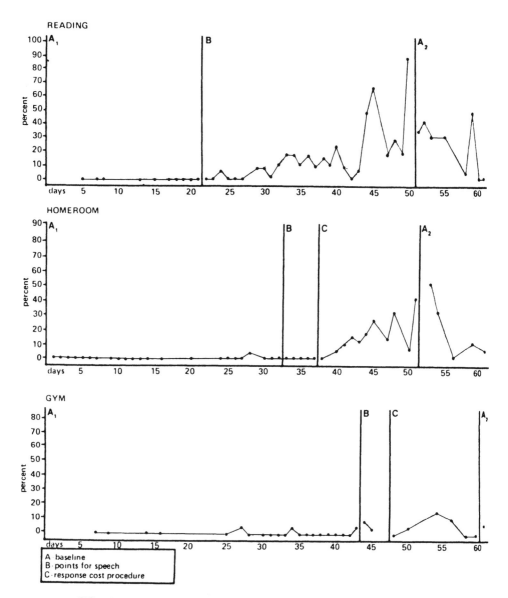

FIG. 5.25. The subject's spontaneous speech to peers per 5-minute periods in the three classes measured: reading class, homeroom, and gym class. (Source: Griffith, E. E., Schnelle, J. F., McNees, M. P., Bissinger, C., & Huff, T. M. Elective mutism in a first grader: The remediation of a complex behavioral problem. *Journal of Abnormal Child Psychology*, 1975, *3*, 127–134. Reproduced by permission.)

teachers also reported that she demonstrated not only verbal compliance but also spontaneous speech. Unfortunately, a 2-year follow-up found the girl verbally noncompliant.

Subject 3 failed to make any verbal response during baseline (5 days) and participated inconsistently in nonverbal activities. During the treatment phase, the boy complied consistently with a series of commands for nonverbal behavior and was reinforced with praise, tokens, and special privileges. Because various positive contingencies were ineffective in eliciting speech, a contingency was arranged in which all students were required to stay in the classroom during recess, at lunch, and during free time until the child asked to be released. The child was allowed to say "yes" if he wanted to go to recess. On the 5th day of the 2nd week, he responded and was released and reinforced. The authors also implemented generalization procedures. At the completion of the program, the child complied 100% of the time with the teacher and aide. Over the course of the year, the child continued to respond verbally to an increasing number of contacts and situations. Follow-up a year later suggested that the child made 17 verbal compliance responses (plus two spontaneous comments) during a 30-minute period.

As the authors note, "Because few experimental controls were built into the procedures of this study, conclusions must be considered tenuous and subject to scientific verification [p. 252]." The report does suggest that a package program approach seems like a worthwhile area of therapeutic programming.

Some researchers have focused their attention on the issue of generalization in the treatment of selective mutism (Appelman, Allen, & Turner, 1975; Sanok & Striefel, 1979). Appelman et al. (1975) assessed the feasibility of conducting speech-conditioning sessions within a preschool classroom and examined the process of transfer of learned verbalizations from those sessions to classroom free time. The child was a nonverbal, 4½-year-old boy whose lack of speech was a major concern to his parents and teachers. Apparently, the boy had verbalized normally at the age of 2 years but became totally nonverbal by age 3. However, it was noted that he had produced the word *okay* in the classroom at the time the study was begun.

Conditioning sessions were held in the preschool classroom. During these sessions, crackers were used as reinforcers. Four phases were programmed in the study. In Phase I a preassessment was made of the child's verbalizations during the classroom free period (the first 30 minutes of the morning). During Phase II daily speech sessions were conducted in the classroom. Assessments of verbalizations continued as in Phase I. In Phase III, the experimenter trained teachers in the techniques employed during speech sessions. Teachers were also instructed to cue the subject during free time to facilitate generalization. In Phase IV the teachers attempted to bring verbal behavior under control of the natural environment by requiring verbal responses for various desired objects in the classroom.

Results for the speech sessions are reported in Fig. 5.26. They appear to indicate that the child learned the six target words in sessions conducted in the

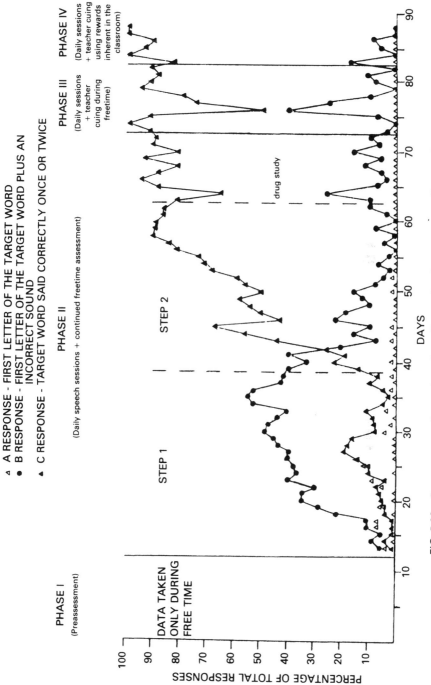

FIG. 5.26. Response to cues in speech sessions. (Source: Appelman, K., Allen, K. E., & Turner, K. D. The conditioning of language in a nonverbal child conducted in a special education classroom. *Journal of Speech and Hearing Disorders*, 1975, *40*, 3–12. Reproduced by permission.)

△ A RESPONSE - FIRST LETTER OF THE TARGET WORD
● B RESPONSE - FIRST LETTER OF THE TARGET WORD PLUS AN
　　　　　　　 INCORRECT SOUND
▲ C RESPONSE - TARGET WORD SAID CORRECTLY ONCE OR TWICE

PHASE I
(Preassessment)

DATA TAKEN
ONLY DURING
FREE TIME

PHASE II
(Daily speech sessions + continued freetime assessment)

STEP 1

STEP 2

drug study

PHASE III
(Daily sessions
+ teacher
cuing during
freetime)

PHASE IV
(Daily sessions
+ teacher cuing
using rewards
inherent in the
classroom)

PERCENTAGE OF TOTAL RESPONSES

DAYS

classroom. By Day 57, the child correctly imitated 85% of the experimenter's cues. For the remaining 31 session days, the percentage of correct responses remained at 80% or above on all but 3 days. Whereas correct responses were low (e.g., less than 15% of the total responses per session) during Step 1 of the conditioning process (Phase II), when the criterion for reinforcement was changed to a C response during Step 2, the percentage of correct responses steadily increased to criterion (at least 85% responding). Moreover, whereas A responses (the first phoneme of the target word) were at a low rate throughout the study, the daily percentage of B responses (the first phoneme of the word plus any sound but the correct one) demonstrated an increase during Step 1, when they and all other vocalizations were reinforced. During Step 2, when B responses were ignored, they dropped to a low rate.

Figure 5.27, which shows the number of cues given to the child by teachers, indicates that the daily number of cues was quite variable until Day 67. No cues were presented on 57% of the days, and teachers cued the child three times or less on 80% of the days. During Phase III, teachers presented five or more daily cues 100% of the time. The child's rate of responding increased from an average of 9% during the previous phases to an average of 72%. During Phase IV, when teachers continued daily cuing, correct responding was at an average of 57%.

Figure 5.28 represents data on spontaneous, noncued whole words emitted by the child. Note that during Step 2 (Phase II) of the therapy sessions, when a whole-word response was the criterion for reinforcement, spontaneous words during free time jumped to an average of 5.0 words per day. Although generalization was occurring, it was inconsistent. In an attempt to increase the child's spontaneous speech, a new contingency was introduced on Day 67 that involved the use of consistent cuing during free time. During Phase III, the subject averaged 5.5 words per day, and during Phase IV, the number of spontaneous words increased to an average of 6.2 per day.

Although the study allows some modest statements about the treatment and generalization components, the progressive design confound (i.e., A–B–$C_1$–$C_2$–D–E) makes between-phase comparisons difficult. Moreover, a "drug study" prior to Phase III further complicates interpretative statements.

Sanok and Striefel (1979) combined positive reinforcement and response cost to establish four classes of verbal responding in an 11-year-old girl who had been selectively mute for approximately 6 years. For approximately 18 months, a variety of interventions had been attempted, including positive reinforcement procedures in the classroom setting, but without success. In the present intervention, the five classes of target behaviors included yes–no answers, single-word responses, multiword responses, reading sentences, and verbally prompted speech. A pool of target stimuli (30 total items) were also selected for each of these classes of target behaviors at a level suitable to the subject's skills level. The program was evaluated in two experiments. In Experiment 1, a multiple baseline design with probes was used across people, settings, and verbal re-

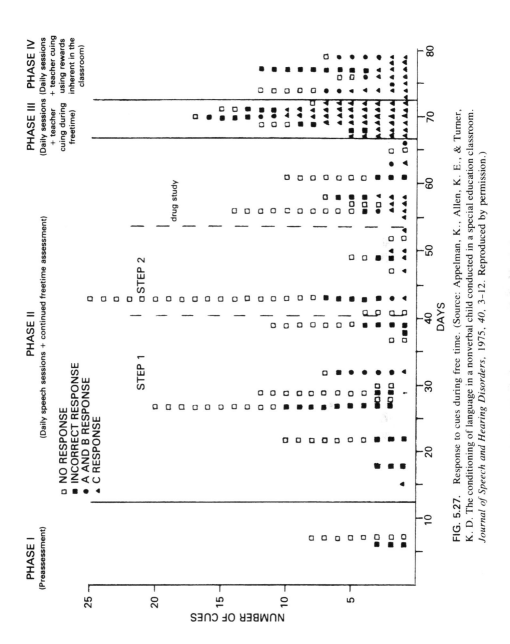

FIG. 5.27. Response to cues during free time. (Source: Appelman, K., Allen, K. E., & Turner, K. D. The conditioning of language in a nonverbal child conducted in a special education classroom. *Journal of Speech and Hearing Disorders*, 1975, *40*, 3–12. Reproduced by permission.)

sponse classes to assess the generalization of verbal responding. Figure 5.29 shows the condensed flowchart of the verbal response training program that was used across each class of target behavior. Figure 5.30 shows the summary of the subject's responses to the target items for Trainer 1 during baseline and treatment conditions at the child center. As Figure 5.30 illustrates, the combined positive reinforcement was successful across each class of target behavior and dramatically increased the subject's verbal responding to Trainer 1 in both training settings for four of the five target behavior classes. Table 5.3 shows that the successive training of one yes–no item, two single-word items, six multiword items, and no reading-sentences items in Setting 1 was necessary to produce verbal response to the remaining items for these classes of target behavior in the presence of Trainer 1. Verbal responding fully generalized from Setting 1 to Setting 2, with the exception of the single-word class of target behavior, in which a single item had to be trained in order to reach the performance criterion.

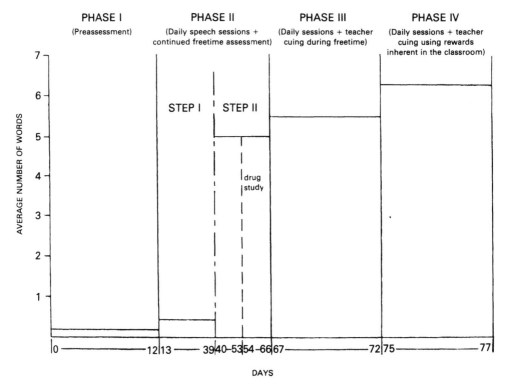

FIG. 5.28.   Spontaneous whole words during free time. (Source: Appelman, K., Allen, K. E., & Turner, K. D. The conditioning of language in a nonverbal child conducted in a special education classroom. *Journal of Speech and Hearing Disorders*, 1975, *40*, 3–12. Reproduced by permission.)

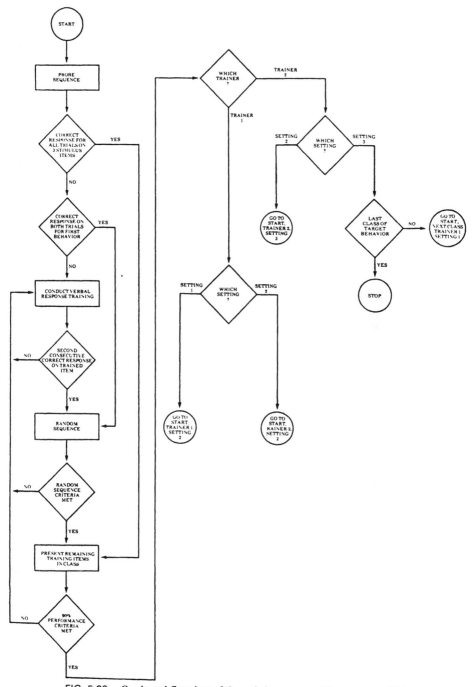

FIG. 5.29. Condensed flowchart of the verbal response training program. With successful completion of training on a class of target behavior across two settings for both trainers, the subject continued training by returning to the beginning of the sequence shown on the first flowchart. Training continued with the next class of target behavior. (Source: Sanok, R. L., & Striefel, S. Elective mutism: Generalization of verbal responding across people and settings. *Behavior Therapy*, 1979, *10*, 357–371. Reproduced by permission.)

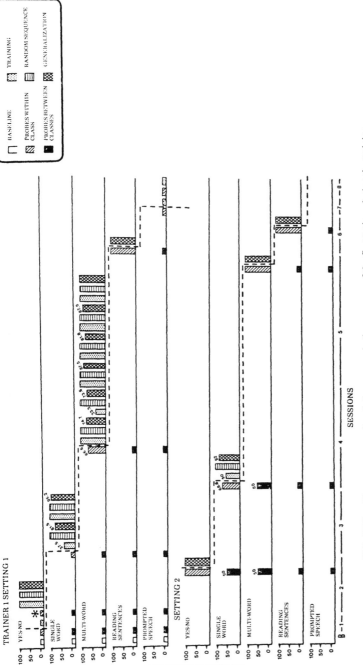

**FIG. 5.30.** The percentage of verbal responses in the presence of the first trainer during the training sequence across the five classes of target behavior in two training settings (Setting 1 and Setting 2). Percentages are based on 10 items per class for baseline, 6 items for probes within a class, 2 items per class for probes between classes, and 6 items for the random sequence. Training and generalization percentages were based on a variable number of items (see text). Asterisk refers to a probe sequence that should not have been conducted. The dashed line indicates the point within a class where training was initiated or would have been initiated if the subject had not met the probe criteria. (Source: Sanok, R. L., & Striefel, S. Elective mutism: Generalization of verbal responding across people and settings. *Behavior Therapy*, 1979, *10*, 357–371. Reproduced by permission.)

TABLE 5.3
Number of Trained Items per Class of Target Behavior and Number
of Items to Which Generalization Occurred After Training*

| | Trainer 1 | | | | Trainer 2 | | | |
| | Setting 1 | | Setting 2 | | Setting 2 | | Setting 3 | |
| Class of Target Behavior | $T^a$ | $G^b$ | T | G | T | G | T | G |
|---|---|---|---|---|---|---|---|---|
| Yes–No | $1(50)^c$ | 29 | 0 | 30 | 1(2) | 29 | 0 | 30 |
| Single-word | 2(10) | 28 | 1(4) | $26^d$ | 0 | 30 | — | — |
| Multiword | 6(16) | 24 | 0 | 30 | — | — | — | — |
| Reading sentences | 0 | 30 | 0 | 30 | — | — | — | — |
| Prompted speech | 1(100) | 0 | 0 | 0 | — | — | — | — |

$^a$"T" refers to items trained.

$^b$"G" refers to generalization items.

$^c$Number of training trials.

$^d$Although all 30 stimulus items were not learned in this setting, the subject did meet a criterion of 90%.

*Source: Sanok and Striefel (1979).

Figure 5.31 shows a summary of the subject's responses to the target stimuli for Trainer 2 under baseline and treatment conditions at the center. Subsequent to meeting criterion for yes–no responses in Settings 1 and 2 for Trainer 1 (Session 2), probes conducted by Trainer 2 indicated increases in yes–no answers (83.3%), multiword responses (100%), and reading sentences (100%). Therefore, training effects generalized to Trainer 2 as a result of previous training of yes–no answers by Trainer 1 in Setting 2.

Experiment 2 used an abbreviated stimulus-fading procedure to transfer verbal responding to strangers and a teacher. Results reported in Fig. 5.32 provide a summary of the subject's responses during the fading procedure in the three settings. Although the first introduction of Stranger 1 into the situation decreased verbal responding to 50% and resulted in a return to the original condition (Trainer 1 alone), which then reinstated verbal responding, the remaining data show that the subject generally responded correctly during the transfer of stimulus control from Trainer 1 to Stranger 1, and from Stranger 1 to Stranger 2. Figure 5.32 also shows the subject's responses during the fading procedures in the child's home and at her school. Whereas the subject emitted correct verbal responses to the sample stimuli presented during the transfer of stimulus control from Trainer 1 to Stranger 3, and from Trainer 1 to the teacher, the child did not show the initial decrement in verbal responding that was apparent with the introduction of Stranger 1 during the transfer training at the child center. This study addresses the manner by which treatment effects are produced across settings with selective mutism. A 10-month follow-up indicated that the treatment gains remained durable. Concomitant improvements in academic areas were noted.

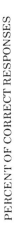

PERCENT OF CORRECT RESPONSES

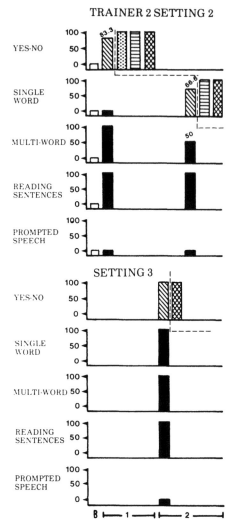

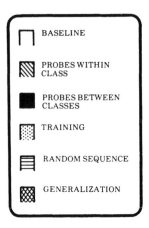

FIG. 5.31. The percentage of verbal responses in the presence of the second trainer during the training sequence across five classes of target behavior in two training settings (Setting 2 and Setting 3). Percentages were based on 10 items per class for baseline, 6 items for probes within a class, 2 items per class for probes between classes, and 6 items for the random sequence. Percentages for training and generalization were based on a variable number of items (see text).

The dashed lines indicates the point within a class where training was initiated or would have been initiated if the subject had not met probe criteria. Sessions 1 and 2 for the second trainer correspond to Sessions 3 and 5 for the first trainer. (Source: Sanok, R. L., & Striefel, S. Elective mutism: Generalization of verbal responding across people and settings. *Behavior Therapy*, 1979, *10*, 357–371. Reproduced by permission.)

112

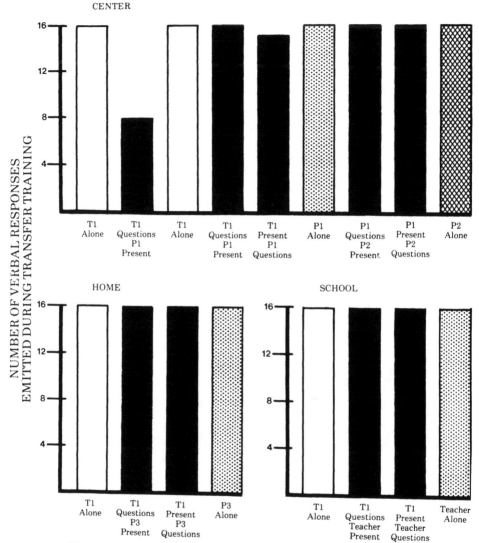

FIG. 5.32. The top graph shows the number of sample verbal responses that occurred during a one-session transfer of training procedure with the first trainer (T1) and two adult strangers (P1 and P2) at the child center. The bottom graphs show the number of sampled verbal responses that occurred during transfer of training procedures to an adult stranger (P3) in the home and to a teacher at school. The maximum number of responses possible in each step was 16. (Source: Sanak, R. L., & Striefel, S. Elective mutism: Generalization of verbal responding across people and settings. *Behavior Therapy,* 1979, *10,* 357–371. Reproduced by permission.)

## Combined Settings

In a novel report, Dowrick and Hood (1978) exposed two selectively mute children, aged 5 and 6 years, to videotape films of themselves that created illusions of appropriate behaviors in target settings. The method employed was developed out of the technique of "self-modeling," which was first described by Creer and Miklich (1970). Self-modeling may be defined as *the behavior change that results from self-observation on videotapes that show only desired target behaviors.* In the present study, the technique arose out of successive failed attempts to use videotape replay techniques for the purpose. The two children were shown short films (5½ minutes) of one or the other of themselves three times a week and were evaluated in a multiple baseline fashion using data recorded by independent observers in class and home settings. The films were made by the suitable editing of target situations recorded in class, together with appropriate responses by the children recorded in their homes where verbal responses occurred freely.

An examination of Fig. 5.33 shows that the rate of classroom talking increased for both subjects following film observation. As Fig. 5.33 illustrates, there is an effect for the self-film for each child, whereas there was no evidence of an effect for the peer film. The magnitude of change was greater for Subject 2. Also, there were only slight changes evident for Subject 1 during her first phase of exposure to her own film. The authors note that she might have benefited more if she had been allowed a more extended treatment (i.e., a longer exposure to films or longer phases). Follow-up observations after 6 months indicated that gains had been maintained.

Dowrick and Hood (1978) indicate that their results appear to be coherent with Bandura's (1977a) "self-efficacy" theory. In this regard, selective mutism is a disorder in which the client already possesses sufficient knowledge and skills to respond effectively, yet does not do so. Bandura (1977a) describes this as an insufficient "perceived self-efficacy" and describes therapeutic change as "partly the acquisition of coping skills and also the acquisition of a self-belief that one can successfully execute the behavior required [p. 193]." Thus, it could be predicted that in situations in which the client lacks the self-belief but not the coping skills, a self-model would be more effective than a peer model.

Jackson and Wallace (1974) treated a 15-year-old severely disturbed girl for aphonia. Specifically, they targeted voice loudness increases in a classroom setting. Due to the extensive nature of the girl's withdrawal, she was conditioned in a laboratory setting and received tokens for speaking loudly enough to operate a voice-operated relay. Conditioning at first consisted of saying 100 monosyllabic words, with the possibility of reinforcement on each word. Thereafter, the girl was required to say a polysyllabic word and, finally, five or six words per token. The loudness data for the "shaping" sessions in mean decibels per word are presented in Fig. 5.34. The girl's decibel level is indicated relative

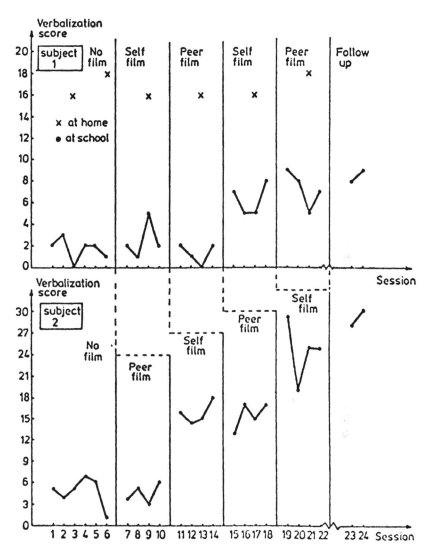

FIG. 5.33. Rate of classroom talking by both subjects following film observation. (Source: Dowrick, P. W., & Hood, M. Transfer of talking behaviors across settings using faked films. In E. L. Glynn & S. S. McNaughton (Eds.), *Proceedings of New Zealand Conference for Research in Applied Behavior Analysis*. Auckland: University of Auckland Press, 1978.

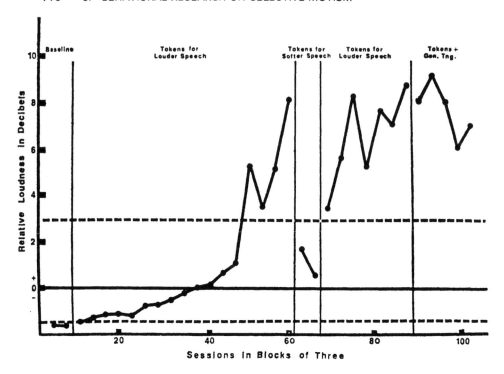

FIG. 5.34.  Results of the "shaping" sessions, in blocks of three sessions per data point. The data are shown in relation to the average loudness of the subject's peers in this setting (zero point on the ordinate). The range for these subjects is shown by the dashed line. After baseline, tokens were given for meeting a loudness or softness criteria. Additional procedures were used in the final experimental phase to ensure behavior change in the classroom. (Source: Jackson, D. A., & Wallace, R. F. The modification and generalization of voice loudness in a fifteen-year-old retarded girl. *Journal of Applied Behavior Analysis,* 1974, 7, 461–471. Copyright by the Society for Experimental Analysis of Behavior. Reproduced by permission.)

to a zero point, which is the mean decibel level produced by her classmates in the "shaping" setting. The range of the voice loudness of Alice's classmates in this setting is shown by broken lines.

Lab generalization checks are presented in Fig. 5.35. Of approximately 1100 words spoken by the girl in each of these sessions, 50-word samples were analyzed from the beginning, middle, and end of each session. Although increases in voice loudness were never differentially reinforced in this setting, loudness gradually improved such that by the end of the experiment, the intensity of her voice was well within the range of intensities of her classmates.

The authors also discovered that early in the "tokens for louder speech" phase, the girl was reading more loudly at the beginning of the "lab generalization checks" than later in those sessions. Thus, immediately after the "shaping" session, as the "lab generalization check" began, the girl spoke louder than she did a few minutes later. This temporary effect is presented in Fig. 5.36. Each of the four lines in this figure indicates combined data gathered over a series of successive sessions to show the general progress of the girl's voice loudness as a "lab generalization check" progressed at four different points in the experimental procedure (see Fig. 5.34 for the specific sessions represented).

Finally, data from the "classroom generalization checks" are shown in Fig. 5.37. Again, the average voice intensity is indicated by the solid line at the zero

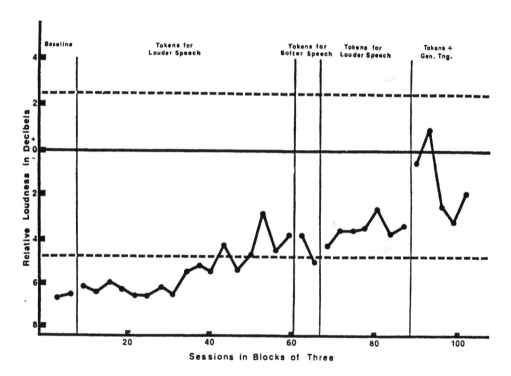

FIG. 5.35.   Results of the "lab generalization checks" in blocks of three sessions per data point. The data are shown in relation to the average loudness of the subject's peers in this setting (zero point on the ordinate). The range for these subjects is shown by the dashed lines. No reinforcement contingencies were used in these checks. (Source: Jackson, D. A., & Wallace, R. F. The modification and generalization of voice loudness in a fifteen-year-old retarded girl. *Journal of Applied Behavior Analysis,* 1974, *7,* 461–471. Copyright by the Society for Experimental Analysis of Behavior. Reproduced by permission.)

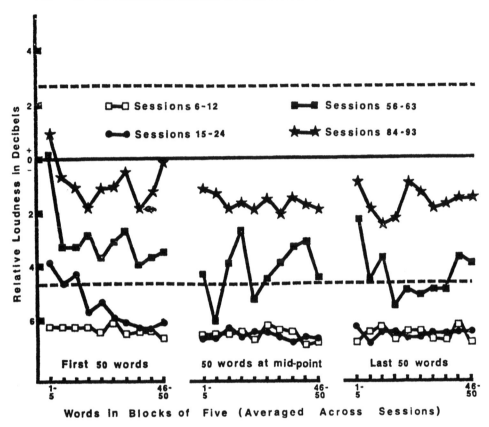

FIG. 5.36.   Relative loudness of Alice's voice as "lab generalization checks" progressed at four different points in the experimental procedure. Each data line represents combined data taken over a series of successive sessions. The average loudness of successive blocks of five words was determined from the data for these combined sessions and is represented here for the first 50 words spoken, the 50 words at the halfway point of the sessions, and for 50 words at the end of the sessions. (Source: Jackson, D. A., & Wallace, R. F. The modification and generalization of voice loudness in a fifteen-year-old retarded girl. *Journal of Applied Behavior Analysis,* 1974, *7,* 461–471. Copyright by the Society for Experimental Analysis of Behavior. Reproduced by permission.)

point on the ordinate, and the range is indicated by the two broken lines. Although there appeared to be little or no generalization from the "shaping" sessions to the "classroom" sessions during the first three experimental phases, the procedures used in "tokens plus generalization training" produced a fairly immediate increase in voice loudness. The authors noted that during the next year, improvements in both voice loudness and social behaviors (e.g., smiling, playing with others, initiating verbal interactions) were quite dramatic.

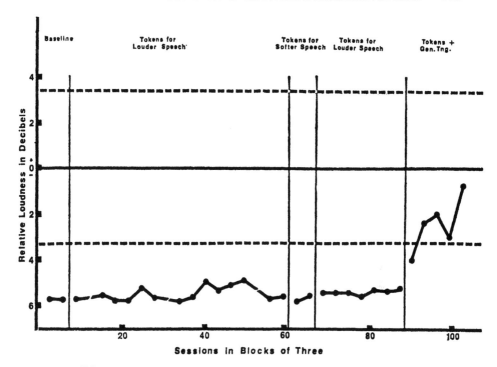

FIG. 5.37.    Results of the "classroom generalization checks" shown in blocks of three sessions per data point. The data are shown in relation to the average loudness of the subject's peers in this setting (zero point on the ordinate). The range for these subjects is shown by the dashed lines. No reinforcement contingencies for loud speech were used until the "tokens plus generalization training" phase. (Source: Jackson, D. A., & Wallace, R. F. The modification and generalization of voice loudness in a fifteen-year-old retarded girl. *Journal of Applied Behavior Analysis*, 1974, *7*, 461–471. Copyright by the Society for Experimental Analysis of Behavior. Reproduced by permission.)

Austad, Sininger, and Stricklin (1980) reported the successful treatment of a 7½ year old girl who spoke only to her mother, but never to other family members, peers, or teachers. Treatment was carried out in the home and clinic settings. In the home, the parents were to eliminate negative statements about talking and to positively reinforce speaking out loud. Treatment in the clinic setting conducted by two therapists lasted 90 minutes per day, 5 days per week for 2 weeks; every other day for 60 minutes for 1 week; and once more for 60 minutes. Across four phases of treatment various procedures were implemented including tangible reinforcement (M & M's), token reinforcement, shaping (Phase I), fading added to these (Phase II), elimination of tangibles (M & M's), food reinforcement, (Phase III), and a contingency with a pet rabbit (Phase IV). The treatment was reported to be successful and to have generalized. The parents reported that she spoke to neighborhood friends and peers at school. The child also responded appropriately to adult verbal requests. A three month follow-up was also positive on these dimensions.

## SUMMARY OF BEHAVIORAL RESEARCH REPORTS

Generally, behavioral interventions focusing on selective mutism have shown a positive pattern of results. Behavioral researchers have intervened across clinic (e.g., Norman & Broman, 1970; Reed, 1963; Shaw, 1971), school (e.g., Bauermeister & Jemail, 1975; Calhoun & Koenig, 1973; Piersel & Kratochwill, in press) and combined settings, such as clinic, school, or other natural settings (Conrad et al., 1974; Williamson et al., 1977b; Wulbert et al., 1973). A variety of intervention procedures have been employed, with relatively straightforward reinforcement (social and tangible) being the most common procedures used. In many of the cases, shaping and fading procedures were presumably necessary to elicit speech. This is likely due to the fact that speech was at zero frequency in all but a few select settings (e.g., home) and had been so for months and, in some cases, years. There appears to be some increase in the number of package treatment programs that include several independent therapeutic procedures and techniques.

Although many authors presumably found it necessary to combine various treatment procedures (reinforcement, shaping, time-out) into treatment packages to effect desired change, the specific contribution of the components remains unknown. Where follow-up was assessed, many researchers reported maintenance of the therapeutic effects. Some generalization was noted, but this remains a problem area—both in terms of assessment and programming.

Perhaps the major limitation of the vast majority of the behavioral reports is the failure to employ credible design and assessment procedures. This finding must prompt a word of caution regarding the efficacy of various programs. Specific issues relating to major methodological concerns are presented in Chapter 6.

# 6 Methodological Review and Recommendations

Generally, the results reported in the psychodynamic (Chapter 3) and behavior therapy (Chapter 5) literature present a positive pattern in the treatment of selective mutism. The two contrasting approaches to treatment of selective mutism present the option of comparing them on various outcome measures. There has been increased interest over the years in comparing behavior therapy with traditional or verbal psychotherapies, and it is not uncommon to find this characterized as a race (see Kazdin & Wilson, 1978, for a review). However, there are problems in making simple comparisons between these two fields of therapeutic endeavor. Kazdin and Wilson (1978) listed some common, but questionable, assumptions of this comparative approach:

1. The terms "behavior therapy" and "psychotherapy" refer to well-defined, internally consistent sets of concepts and readily reproducible operations that can be usefully compared to each other or to something labeled "routine treatment."
2. Generally applicable and standardized measures exist (e.g., clinical ratings) that can be used to evaluate the relative efficacy of these alternative forms of therapy.
3. Treatment outcome can be evaluated in terms of qualitative concepts such as "cure," "relapse," and "remission."
4. Outcome studies can be evaluated in a summary, qualitative fashion as showing that a particular therapy is significantly superior to, inferior to, or no different from an alternative therapy, and,
5. A balance sheet or box score can be derived in which diverse studies are assigned to one of these discrete categories and the resultant cumulative totals meaningfully compared [p. 105].

Kazdin and Wilson (1978) were primarily referring to comparative treatment outcome studies. Nevertheless, their criticism of these five commonly uncritically accepted assumptions applies to the literature reviewed here. The critical issue is which treatment administered by which therapist is most effective for what problem in which patient. Central to this analysis is specificity and operational precision in applied therapeutic research.

The literature on selective mutism raises a number of concerns that need careful elaboration. A significant number of concerns remain unanswered in both the psychodynamic and behavior therapy literature that require careful examination if treatment and future research strategies are to be useful. Because the $N = 1$ research strategy appears to be the major option in conducting research in this area, both therapeutic models are discussed in the context of the methodological issues involved in this form of investigation. Of course, comparisons between the two paradigms are made where appropriate.

This chapter extends the methodological critique offered by the author and his associates previously (Kratochwill et al., 1979). It draws from this earlier review as well as from recent methodological and assessment issues raised in the review of psychotherapy and behavior therapy (Bergin & Suinn, 1975; Games-Schwartz, Hadley, & Strupp, 1978; Kazdin & Wilson, 1978; Krasner, 1971). The chapter raises methodological and assessment issues and offers some recommendations for future research.

## METHODOLOGICAL AND ASSESSMENT CONSIDERATIONS

The methodological and assessment issues in applied research have proliferated in recent years. A growing body of literature has elucidated the important issues that must be considered in drawing conclusions from a body of existing research and the conduct of future research in a particular area. Several of the relevant dimensions to be considered when evaluating the research in the area of selective mutism are presented in Tables 6.1 and 6.2. Table 6.1 presents an overview of the psychodynamic studies offering descriptive and/or treatment data on selective mutism. Table 6.2 provides an overview of the behavior therapy studies in the area. The more conventional descriptive and methodological issues are listed in these tables, but a more extensive discussion is presented in this chapter. The issues to be considered include: outcome measures, generalization, definition of selective mutism, research design, systematic treatment evaluation strategies, direct assessment, outcome evaluation criteria, and social validation.

### Outcome Measures

A major methodological problem in the research on selective mutism, and particularly in the psychodynamic area, is the lack of adequate measures of treatment outcome. Several specific issues can be identified. In the case of the

## TABLE 6.1
### Overview of Intrapsychic Treatment Studies on Selective Mutism

| Author(s) | N | Setting(s) | Major Intervention Technique(s) | Sex of Subjects | S Ages | Design | Systematic Variation of Treatment | Multiple Measures | Observer Agreement Assessed | Generalization Measures | Follow-Up |
|---|---|---|---|---|---|---|---|---|---|---|---|
| Adams (1970) | 1 | clinic | psychotherapy | male | 6 | case study | No | No | No | No | Yes (unspecified) |
| Adams & Glasner (1954) | 1 | clinic | psychotherapy | female | 4–4 | case study | No | No | No | No | Yes (unspecified) |
| | 1 | clinic | psychotherapy | male | 4–6 | study | No | No | No | No | No |
| | 2 twins | clinic | psychotherapy | male | 9–6 | study | No | No | No | No | Yes (11 + 12 yrs) |
| Browne, Wilson, & Laybourne (1963) | 1 | home | psychotherapy (family) | male | 6 | case study | No | No | No | No | No |
| Chetnik (1973) | 1 | clinic | psychotherapy | female | 6–5 | case study | No | No | No | No | No |
| Elles (1962) | 1 | hospital | psychotherapy | male | 3 | case study | No | No | No | No | No |
| Elson, Pearson, Jones, & Schumacker (1965) | 1 | clinic | psychotherapy | female | 7–6 | case study | No | No | No | Yes | Yes (6 mos) |
| | 3 | clinic | milieu therapy | 3 females | 7–10 | case study | No | No | No | No | Yes (to 5 yrs) |
| Halpern, Hammond, & Cohen (1971) | 1 | clinic-natural environment | (quasi) behavioral | male | 7 | case study | No | No | No | No | No |
| | 2 | clinic-natural environment | (quasi) behavioral | females | 6½ | case study | No | No | No | No | No |
| | | | | | 6½ | | No | No | No | No | No |
| Howard (1963) | 1 | hospital | art therapy | male | 8 | case study | No | No | No | No | No |
| Kaplan & Escoll (1973) | 1 | hospital | psychotherapy | female | 15 | case study | No | No | No | No | Yes (5 mos) |

*(continued)*

**TABLE 6.1** *(continued)*

| Author(s) | N | Setting(s) | Major Intervention Technique(s) | Sex of Subjects | S Ages | Design | Systematic Variation of Treatment | Multiple Measures | Observer Agreement Assessed | Generalization Measures | Follow-Up |
|---|---|---|---|---|---|---|---|---|---|---|---|
| Kass, Gillman, Mattis, Klugman, & Jacobson (1967) | 1 | hospital | psychotherapy | female | 17 | case study | No | No | No | No | No |
| | 1 | clinic | psychotherapy | female | 6–5 | case study | No | No | No | No | Yes (unspecified) |
| Koch (1976) | 15 | hospital | psychotherapy | 10 males 5 females | 8–21 | case study | No | No | No | No | Yes (X = 4) 8 yr old (X = 9) 14–21 |
| Koch & Goodlund (1973) | 13 | hospital | psychotherapy | 9 males 4 females | 3–6 | case study | No | Yes | No | No | Yes (X = 9 yrs) |
| Landgarten (1975) | 1 | clinic | art therapy | female | 7 | case study | No | No | No | No | Yes (4 mos) |
| Laybourne (1979) | 1 | clinic | psychotherapy | male | 5 | case study | No | No | No | No | Yes (5 yrs) |
| | 1 | hospital | psychotherapy | female | 13 | case study | No | No | No | No | Yes (7 yrs) |
| Mora, Devault, & Schopler (1962) | 2 (twins) | clinic | psychotherapy | females | 13 | case study | No | No | No | No | Yes (unspecified) |
| Morris (1953) | 1 | clinic | psychotherapy | female | 10 | case study | No | No | No | No | Yes (unspecified) |
| | 1 | clinic | | male | 6 | case study | No | No | No | No | No |
| | 1 | clinic | | female | 4 | case study | No | No | No | No | Yes (unspecified) |
| | 1 | clinic | | male | 4 | case study | No | No | No | No | Yes (1 yr) |
| | 1 | clinic | | female | 9 | case study | No | No | No | No | No |
| | 1 | clinic | | male | unspecified | case study | No | No | No | No | No |
| Parker, Olsen, & Throckmorton (1960) | 27 ex post (single-case studies) | school | social casework with teachers, parents and child | 13 females 14 males | unspecified elementary | case study | No | No | No | No | No |

| Study | N | Setting | Treatment | Sex | Age | Type | | | | | | |
|---|---|---|---|---|---|---|---|---|---|---|---|---|
| Pustrom & Speers (1964) | 1 | hospital | psychotherapy | male | 8 | case study | No | No | No | No | No | No |
| | 1 | hospital | | male | 8 | case study | No | No | No | No | No | No |
| | 1 | hospital | | female | 8 | case study | No | No | No | No | No | No |
| Rigby (1929) | 1 | clinic | psychotherapy | male | 6 | case study | No | No | No | No | No | No |
| Ruzicka & Sackin (1974) | 1 | hospital | psychotherapy | female | 9 | case study | No | No | No | No | No | No |
| Salfield, Lond, & Dusseldorf (1950) | 1 | clinic | psychotherapy | male | 7 | case study | No | No | No | No | No | No |
| Silverman & Powers (1970) | 5 | clinic | psychotherapy | 3 males 2 females | 13,14,4 7,12 | case study | No | No | No | No | No | Yes (4, 6 mos or unspecified) |
| Smayling (1959) | 1 | clinic | speech therapy | male | 6 | case | No | No | No | No | No | No |
| | 1 | clinic | | female | 5–6 | study | No | No | No | No | No | No |
| | 1 | clinic | | female | 5–6 | case | No | No | No | No | No | No |
| | 1 | clinic | | female | 6 | study | No | No | No | No | No | No |
| | 1 | clinic | | female | 6 | case | No | No | No | No | No | No |
| | 1 | clinic | | male | 10 | study | No | No | No | No | No | No |
| | | | | male | 6 | case | No | No | No | No | No | No |
| Strait (1958) | 1 | school | speech therapy | male | 6 | case study | No | No | No | No | No | No |
| Wright (1968) | 24 single cases | clinic | psychotherapy | 7 males 17 females | 5–25% 6–25% 7–34% 8–8% 9–8% | case study | No | No | No | No | No | Yes (6 mos to 7 yrs) |

## TABLE 6.2
### Overview of Behavioral Treatment Studies on Selective Mutism

| Author(s) | N | Setting(s) | Major Intervention Technique(s) | Sex of Subjects | S Ages | Design | Systematic Variation of Treatment | Multiple Measures | Observer Agreement Assessed | Generalization Measures | Follow-Up |
|---|---|---|---|---|---|---|---|---|---|---|---|
| Adkins (1975) | 1 | school | time-out, reinforcement | female | 6.0 | case study | No | No | No | No | No |
| Appelman, Allen, & Turner (1975) | 1 | preschool | reinforcement, shaping, cuing | male | 4.6 | ABC, C₂DE | Yes | Yes | Yes | Yes | No |
| Austad, Sininger, & Stricklin (1980) | 1 | home & client | positive reinforcement, shaping, fading, tokens, contingency contracting | female | 7.5 | case study | No | No | No | No | Yes (3 mos) |
| Bauermeister & Jemail (1975) | 1 | school | reinforcement | male | 8.0 | case study | Yes | Yes | Yes | Yes | Yes (1 yr) |
| Bednar (1974) | 1 | school | reinforcement, shaping | male | 10 | case study | No | No | No | Yes | Yes (2 yrs) |
| Blake & Moss (1967) | 1 | clinic | imitation, shaping, reinforcement | female | 4 | AB | Yes | Yes | No | Yes | No |
| Brison (1966) | 1 | school | time-out, reinforcement | male | kindergarten | case study | No | No | No | No | Yes (3 yrs) |
| Calhoun & Koenig (1973) | 8 | school | reinforcement | unspecified | 5-8 | AB | Yes | No | Yes | No | Yes (1 yr) |
| Colligan, Colligan, & Dilliard (1977) | 1 | school | reinforcement, contingency mgmt. | male | 11 | case study | No | No | No | Yes | Yes (1 yr) |
| Conrad, Delk, & Williams (1974) | 1 | home | reinforcement, stimulus fading | female | 11 | case study | Yes | No | No | Yes | Yes (1 yr) |
| Dmitriev & Hawkins (1973) | 1 | school | social reinforcement | female | 9 | case study | Yes | No | No | Yes | Yes (4 yrs) |
| Dowrick & Hood (1978) | 2 | school | self-modeling | male female | 5½ 6 | multiple baseline ABAB | Yes | No | Yes | No | Yes (6 mos) |

| Reference | No. | Type | Setting | Procedures | Sex | No. | Design | | | | | Follow-up |
|---|---|---|---|---|---|---|---|---|---|---|---|---|
| Friedman & Karagan (1973) | 13 | single-case studies | clinic | combination of procedures (see text) | unspecified | | case studies | No | No | No | No | No |
| Griffith, Schnelle, McNees, Bissinger, & Huff (1975) | 1 | | school | reinforcement, response-cost | male | 6 | multiple base line across settings | Yes | Yes | Yes | No | Yes (3 mos) |
| Jackson & Wallace (1974) | 1 | | clinic, laboratory | shaping, reinforcement | female | 15 | ABAB | Yes | Yes | Yes | Yes | Yes (1 yr) |
| Moss & Blake (1970) | 1 | | clinic | reinforcement (psychodynamic) | female | 4 | (A)B | Yes | Yes | No | Yes | No |
| Munford, Reardon, Liberman, & Allen (1976) | 1 | | clinic, home | reinforcement, shaping, instructions, and feedback | female | 17 | combination changing-criterion | Yes | Yes | No | Yes | Yes (41 mos) |
| Nash, Thorpe, Andrews, & Davis (1979) | 3 | | school | prompting, chaining, role playing, reinforcement | female | 5 | AB | Yes | Yes | No | Yes | Yes (2 yrs) |
| | | | | | male | 9 | AB | Yes | Yes | No | Yes | Yes (2 yrs) |
| | | | | | male | 8 | AB | Yes | Yes | Yes (on follow-up) | Yes | Yes (1 yr) |
| Nolan & Pence (1970) | 1 | | home school | fading, reinforcement | female | 10 | case study | No | No | No | Yes | Yes (1 yr) |
| Norman & Broman (1970) | 1 | | clinic | reinforcement | male | 10 | case study | Yes | Yes | No | Yes | Yes (18 mos) |
| Piersel & Kratochwill (in press) | 2 | | school | reinforcement, extinction, mild aversive procedures | male | 5–4 | multiple baseline across situations | Yes | Yes | Yes | Yes | Yes |
| | | | | | female | 4–1 | | | | | | |
| Rasbury (1974) | 1 | | home | systematic desensitization | female | 6 | case study | Yes | No | No | Yes | Yes (1 yr) |
| Reed (1963) | 1 | | clinic | reinforcement (some unspecified procedures) | female | 14 | case study | No | No | No | No | Yes (5 years) |
| | | | clinic | | female | 13 | case study | No | No | No | No | Yes (5 + 10 yrs) |
| | | | clinic | | female | 12 | case study | No | No | No | No | Yes (5 + 11 yrs) |
| | | | clinic | | male | 12 | case study | No | No | No | No | Yes (3 + 11 yrs) |

Continued

**TABLE 6.2—Continued**

| Author(s) | N | Setting(s) | Major Intervention Technique(s) | Sex of Subjects | S Ages | Design | Systematic Variation of Treatment | Multiple Measures | Observer Agreement Assessed | Generalization Measures | Follow-Up |
|---|---|---|---|---|---|---|---|---|---|---|---|
| Reid, Hawkins, Keutzer, McNeal, Phelps, Reid, & Mees (1967) | 1 | clinic | reinforcement, stimulus fading | female | 6 | case study | Yes | No | No | Yes | Yes (2, 3, 4 yrs) |
| Rosenbaum & Kellman (1973) | 1 | school | shaping, social reinforcement | female | 8 | case study | Yes | Yes | No | Yes | Yes (2½ mos) |
| Sanok & Streifel (1979) | 1 | school | reinforcement, response cost | female | 11 | multiple baseline | Yes | Yes | Yes | Yes | No |
| Scott (1977) | 1 | clinic | desensitization, reinforcement | female | 6–5 | B | Yes | No | No | Yes | Yes (3 mos) |
| Semenoff, Park, & Smith (1976) | 1 | school | reinforcement, shaping | male | 4–10 | case study | No | No | No | No | No |
| Shaw (1971) | 1 | clinic | punishment (medication), reinforcement | female | 10½ | case study | No | No | No | No | Yes (1 yr) |
| Sluckin & Jehu (1969) | 1 | home | reinforcement, shaping | female | 4–11 | case study | No | No | No | Yes | Yes (1 yr) |
| Straughan, Potter, & Hamilton (1965) | 1 | special school | reinforcement | male | 14 (retarded) | AB | Yes | Yes | No | No | Yes (1 yr) |

| Study | | Setting | Treatment | Sex | Age | Design | | | | | Follow-up |
|---|---|---|---|---|---|---|---|---|---|---|---|
| Van der Kooy & Webster (1975) | 1 | summer camp | avoidance conditioning, reinforcement, fading | male | 6 | AB | Yes | Yes | No | Yes | Yes (6 mos) |
| Williamson, Sanders, Sewell, Haney, & White (1977a) | 1 | school | shaping w/ modeling, escape and reinforcement, shaping and fading | male | 8 | AB | Yes | No | No | No | Yes (2 wks and 1 year) |
| | 1 | school | shaping w/ modeling, reinforcement and reinforcer sampling, sampling w/ stimulus fading, reinforcement and reinforcement fading | female | 7 | AB | Yes | No | No | No | Yes (1 mo) |
| Williamson, Sewell, Sanders, Haney, & White (1977b) | 1 | clinic, school home | token economy | male | 8 | AB | Yes | No | No | No | Yes (1 yr) |
| | 1 | clinic, school, home | token economy | male | 7 | AB | Yes | Yes | Yes | Yes | Yes (2 wks and 1 yr) |
| Wulbert, Nyman, Snow, & Owen (1973) | 1 | public school, kinder-garten, psychology clinic | stimulus fading, contingency management (time-out) | female | 6 | AB | Yes | Yes | Yes | Yes | No |

psychodynamic approach, a major problem is conceptual. As noted in Chapter 2, a major characteristic of the psychodynamic approach involves an indirect measurement scheme. Mutism was seldom measured by direct behavioral samples; rather, dynamic personality characteristics are inferred from direct or indirect signs. This conceptualization of behavior based on internal dynamics has promoted qualitative rather than quantitative measures (cf. Kazdin & Wilson, 1978), and this is strongly evident in the psychodynamic claims of successful treatment of selective mutism.

In many cases, preassessment and posttherapy assessments of the mute child were made from projective or objective personality tests (e.g., TAT or MMPI) or from global ratings of improvement. In addition to the reliability concerns that this raises (see Hersen & Barlow, 1976), it appears that clinical judgments of personality structures based on interviews, projective, and objective tests have not demonstrated their utility (Kazdin & Wilson, 1978; Mischel, 1968, 1973c). Mischel (1973c) noted:

> The accumulated findings give little support for the utility of clinical judgments even when the judges are expert psychodynamicists, working in clinical contexts and using their favorite techniques. . . . Clinicians guided by concepts about underlying genotypic dispositions have not been able to predict behavior better than have the person's own direct self-report, sample indices of directly relevant past behavior, or demographic variables [p. 254].

Another problem with the traditional assessment procedure is that it typically does not use repeated measurement to examine the pattern of change over the duration of the treatment program. Many of the behavioral case reports likewise did not report continuous measurement to evaluate the program's effectiveness.

*Recommendations.*    Both the psychodynamic and behavior therapy approaches should employ direct measures of speech (and other measures as well) in the natural environment. There are several rationales for this recommendation (cf. Kazdin & Wilson, 1978). First, a direct assessment of speech or lack of speech across situations provides the researcher with specific information on client improvement. The direct assessment procedure is supported by research suggesting that a client is best understood by determining what he or she does (thinks or feels) in various life situations (Mischel, 1973c).

Another rationale for the use of direct measurement is that such measures allow empirical discrimination among different therapeutic procedures. For example, in their work with a selective mutism case, Wulbert et al. (1973) were able to determine that the stimulus-fading procedure was a necessary component of their treatment program and that the time-out contingency for nonresponse was found to facilitate treatment when combined with stimulus fading. Direct and specific behavior measures reduce the subjective bias that characterizes interviews and ratings as outcome measures. Global ratings or impressions can obscure actual treatment outcomes and reflect differences among therapists rather than the client's actual functioning.

Direct behavioral measures should be less affected by bias or other forms of distortion than measures that rely on more global impressions. Kazdin and Wilson (1978) noted that judgments of others on client improvement may have little relation to overt behavioral measures (e.g., Kazdin, 1973a; Schnelle, 1974), and that biases of individuals completing the assessment devices are more likely to enter into global ratings (or impressions) than measures of overt target behavior (Kazdin, 1977a; Kent & Foster, 1977).

Finally, researchers will be able to replicate findings of various treatment programs when direct behavioral measures are employed. This is particularly important in the mutism literature, where systematic replication has been all but nonexistent (cf. Kratochwill et al., 1979). Nevertheless, direct and systematic replication of research procedures seems possible in many clinic settings when measures of select speech are obtained.

A second recommendation is that the direct assessment procedures should be continuous. This will allow both the researcher and those interested in applying the therapeutic procedures to examine patterns or trends in the data. Whereas all the psychodynamic studies failed to use continuous measurement procedures, many of the behavioral studies either reported phase summary measures (e.g., Bauermeister & Jemail, 1975) or no data at all (e.g., Bednar, 1974; Colligan et al., 1977).

Given that direct assessment is the measurement option of choice, what specific devices should be employed? It is beyond the scope of this chapter to review them all, but many useful procedures have recently been presented (e.g., Ciminero et al., 1977; Cone & Hawkins, 1977; Goldfried & Davidson, 1976; Hersen & Barlow, 1976). Particularly useful are procedures that involve direct observational assessment (e.g., Kazdin, 1977a; Kent & Foster, 1977; Kratochwill & Wetzel, 1977) and video- and/or audiotape systems (e.g., Rugh & Schwitzgebel, 1977; Schwitzgebel, 1976).

A third recommendation relates to the use of multiple measures. Davidson and Seidman (1974) observed that no *single* measurement system is inherently valid (see also Campbell & Fiske, 1959). For these reasons, there is increasing recognition that multiple measures of both a subjective and objective nature should be gathered. Three response systems are generally appropriate for multiple assessment (Cone, 1978; Hersen & Barlow, 1976). These include overt behavior (motor), physiological reactions, and self-report (cognitive). Although self-report could not be used in many situations where mutism is occurring, some settings where speech is occurring, such as the home, could be effectively monitored with self-report measures. Such measures, when independently validated, may elucidate certain feared situations or individuals that are partly responsible for maintaining the mutism. Physiological measures seem especially relevant in research and treatment of mutism, but no researchers employed such measures. Such assessment may be especially relevant where medication is employed and/or where strong anxiety is prominent. Perhaps the strongest rationale for multiple measures is that different modalities of assessment may be differentially affected by different therapeutic methods (cf. Kazdin & Wilson, 1978). Presumably, mutism could be related to severe depression or anxiety. In such cases, assessment of affect (self-report) could be combined with direct behavioral measures in other settings.

Given the complexity of the phenomenon labeled "selective mutism," it appears that multiple measures and their degree of correspondence are necessary. Conceptualization of outcome measures on many dimensions (i.e., multivariate) should also help determine the range of pervasiveness of experimental outcomes—that is, the "referent generality" of an intervention as suggested by Snow (1974). Moreover, multiple measures should help elucidate the degree of external validity of experimental outcomes (cf. Cook & Campbell, 1976; Kratochwill, 1978, 1979; Kratochwill & Levin, 1979). In addition, multiple measures should help assess response generalization and discrimination (cf. Kazdin, 1973a). An investigation examining the effectiveness of social reinforcement on mute behavior should also examine other social skills as well as academic performance (Cartledge & Milburn, 1978). Thus, an adequate examination of parents, peers, and other socialization agents, in addition to the usual assessment of experimenters, observers, tests, and so forth, should be performed. This broader approach to assessment should also promote a better image for critics of the behavioral approach who perceive it as a mechanistic therapeutic model (e.g., Laybourne, 1979).

Although only 8% of the psychodynamic and 41% of the behavior therapy research used multiple response measures, future research should actively pursue this direction in the area of selective mutism.

## Generalization

A major methodological consideration in the selective mutism literature relates to the generalizability of the therapeutic results. The research in both psychodynamic and behavior therapy areas has provided some evidence of accomplishing the goal of selective speech in the mute child in some situations. Nevertheless, in the vast majority of cases (i.e., 0% in the psychodynamic and 71% in the behavioral literature), this factor was not even formally *assessed*. Generalization of behavior can be conceptualized as a maintenance and transfer issue. This conceptualization of generalization follows that advanced by Stokes and Baer (1977) (i.e., "generalization is the occurrence of relevant behavior under different, nontraining conditions [across subjects, settings, people, behaviors, and/or time] without the scheduling of the same events in those conditions as had been scheduled in the training conditions" [p. 350]).[1]

Although many of the behavior therapy reports assessed generalization (e.g., Blake & Moss, 1967; Munford et al., 1976), specific programming of this was not planned for in some studies (e.g., Bednar, 1974). Bauermeister and Jemail (1975) argued that the possibility of a failure in generalization of treatment effects was eliminated by applying the treatment program in vivo (i.e., the classroom). Possibly the treatment of the child over two classes facilitated generalization, as well as employing several target responses. Colligan et al. (1977) established a generalization plan based on having staff members engage the child in verbal communication that would require a short verbal response each time they saw the child. Appelman et al. (1975) found that generalization was occurring but that it was inconsistent. Van der Kooy and Webster (1975) programmed generalization to other persons as well as to situations outside the pool. Extra attention was also faded.

Unfortunately, the vast majority of reports did not provide formal assessment of generalization. Also, many of the reports of generalization did not involve direct measures and so were subject to the types of biases already discussed.

*Recommendations.*    As many reports did not assess and actively promote generalization, this should be addressed in future research. The paucity of research reports that actively promoted generalization presumably reflects the lack, until recently, of a generalization technology. In recent years there has been a growing awareness that generalization is not a passive phenomenon, but rather should be actively programmed (e.g., Guess, Keogh, & Sailor, 1978; Kazdin, 1977a,1978a; Marholin, Siegel, & Phillips, 1976; O'Leary & Drabman, 1971; Stokes & Baer, 1977; Wildman & Wildman, 1975). Recently, Stokes and Baer (1977) provided an embryonic technology of generalization that will be useful in future research and treatment of selective mutism. The specific components of this technology are discussed in Chapter 7 and so are not detailed here. Nevertheless, it is advisable that researchers consider procedures that *actively* promote generalization rather than "train and hope" (i.e., train the subject and "hope" that behavior generalizes). The specific tactics offered by Stokes and Baer (1977) provide not only a set of what-to-do treatment possibilities but could also be investigated in future selective mutism intervention programs. Finally, both the generalization tactics and the results should be formally measured by direct means.

---

[1]The Stokes and Baer (1977) conceptualization of generalization differs from that provided by other writers (e.g., Keller & Schoenfeld, 1950; Skinner, 1953).

## Follow-Up Measures and Maintenance

Another methodological issue, follow-up, relates to the measurement of the durability of the treatment program once it is formally discontinued. Within the Stokes and Baer (1977) formulation, maintenance is but one feature in the examination of generalization across time. The majority of the psychodynamic and behavior therapy research on selective mutism includes a follow-up assessment (52% and 59% in each area, respectively). Nevertheless, in the past, behavior therapy has not done exceptionally well in gathering follow-up measures. Cochrane and Sobol (1976), in a review of the contents of four major behavior therapy journals (i.e., *Journal of Applied Behavior Analysis, Journal of Behavior Therapy and Experimental Psychiatry, Behavior Therapy,* and *Behavior Research and Therapy*), found that only 35% of the studies, when follow-ups was necessary, actually included follow-up assessment. Also, less than a third of these follow-up investigations took place more than 6 months after the therapeutic program ended. Likewise, Keeley, Shemberg, and Carbonell (1976) found that between the years 1972 and 1973, only about 12% of the studies in the *Journal of Applied Behavior Analysis, Behavior Therapy,* and *Behavior Research and Therapy* reported follow-up data of more than 6 months' duration. Although many writers have criticized the absence of follow-up in behavior modification research in general (e.g., Cochrane & Sobol, 1976; Keeley, Shemberg, & Carbonell, 1976), one possible reason for the lack of extensive follow-up measurement is that the field is relatively young, with the bulk of research produced since 1970 (cf. Kazdin, 1978b).

With the behavior disorder of selective mutism, the most meaningful estimate of treatment effectiveness can be obtained through accurate and reliable follow-up assessment. However, there are a number of problems in follow-up assessment approaches. First, the psychodynamic approach to follow-up has been based on the quasi-disease model of abnormal behavior, with an emphasis on qualitative concepts such as care, spontaneous remission, or relapse (cf. Bandura, 1969; Kazdin & Wilson, 1978; Ullmann & Krasner, 1975). As Kazdin and Wilson (1978) noted, although such concepts may be appropriately applied to treatment and follow-up of physical disease, they are not generally as useful for measuring behavior changes that are influenced by social psychological variables. When behavior is conceptualized independent of environmental events, and rather through intrapsychic conflicts (see Chapter 2), reoccurrence of the problem may cause the therapist to regard the original treatment as incomplete. Additional therapy then focuses on the same intrapsychic problems presumed to underlie the problem originally.

In contrast to this view, the behavior therapy orientation considers selective mutism as a function of antecedent and consequent environmental events (or cognitive mediating processes) that vary across different situations. This prompts a very different conceptualization of follow-up and maintenance of behavior change. Several issues should be considered (cf. Kazdin & Wilson, 1978). First, different behaviors will vary in the degree to which they are likely to generalize to new situations and to be maintained over time. In the case of mutism, specific programming would seem to be necessary to increase the probability that speech will be maintained. Second, the setting in which the mutism (or newly acquired speaking behavior) occurs may be an extremely important factor in maintenance of the behavior. Finally, variables such as self-control skills (Thoresen & Mahoney, 1974) and expectations of self-efficacy (Bandura, 1977a) may influence the generalization and maintenance of behavior change. There are no reported cases in the behavior therapy literature where self-control strategies were employed in selective treatment, but their use in treatment and in maintenance, particularly after speech is established, seems especially desirable. On the other hand, Dowrick and Hood (1978) used self-modeling strategies to treat selective mutism. They note that it would be predicted that in situations in which the subject lacks the self-belief but not the coping skills, a self-model strategy would be more effective than a peer model.

Another major problem with follow-up measures involves the type of assessment made of the durability of the treatment program (cf. Kratochwill et al., 1979). Many of the measures are characterized by informal interviews, telephone conversations, or generally no direct assessment of the behavior. For example, at the time Munford et al. (1976) were proofreading their mutism manuscript, a phone call was made to the formerly mute child. Williamson et al. (1977a) conducted 2-week and 1-year interviews with teachers to obtain their follow-up data. These represent some of the better follow-up strategies and are to be applauded. However, follow-up measures would include a more direct and formalized measure of the client's functioning whenever possible.

*Recommendations.* Several recommendations for follow-up can be advanced based on previous discussions in the mutism literature (cf. Kratochwill et al., 1979) and the behavior therapy literature in general (cf. Robins, 1979). First, Robins (1979) noted that the essential concept of the follow-up study is that it involves measures at two or more points in time. However, the *kinds* of things measured at these points may be the same or different. For example, in the selective mutism literature, a researcher could examine speech frequency at Time 1 and Time 2. Thus, in this case, the same behaviors are measured twice (or more). In addition, a researcher may measure speech with other behaviors over time, such as social skills, academic performance, and so forth.

Second, within the behavior therapy orientation, measures used to facilitate generalization of behavior can be used to program maintenance of the therapeutic gain (e.g., Stokes & Baer, 1977). Second, future research should obtain a broad range of multiple measures on follow-up. Direct observation of the client under the recording conditions established during the therapeutic program is very desirable (see Williamson et al., 1977b). The use of variables that are identical or similar to those used in the treatment program will enable the researcher to assess the progress of the child on a time continuum using similar measures of performance from one setting to another. Such a procedure would allow assessment in predicting posttreatment performance. Data could also be obtained from individuals knowledgeable of the client's behavior, such as parents, teachers, and peers. However, direct measures of the target behavior will likely represent the best measurement system (Kratochwill et al., 1979).

Finally, frequent follow-up assessment should be made shortly after treatment termination to determine any early relapse trends or problems (cf. Callner, 1975). Follow-up assessment should also be made frequently after treatment termination and less frequently over time. In this way, follow-up assessment could detect problems and thereby allow the application of appropriate ''booster treatments'' to remedy any difficulties. The researcher could also determine if the treatment was effective but failed to maintain change. As Kazdin and Wilson (1978) observed:

> The point is that it is inappropriate to use follow-up information as the sole criterion for a dichotomous all-or-nothing judgment about the success or failure of treatment efficacy. A method that produced an initial effect may represent a useful starting point for the design of a more enduring treatment [p. 133].

Thus, when no other treatment has been effective, a procedure that produces dramatic change should not be dismissed because follow-up suggested little durability.

## Definition of Selective Mutism: The Nature of the Problem

*The Psychodynamic Model.*   A conventional approach to defining mutism lies in the psychodynamic model of abnormal behavior. For example, the various writers in the psychodynamic area appear to account for mutism somewhat differently. Whereas some writers take the position that the primary difficulty appears in the oral stage of psychosexual development and is intermittently related to difficulties in object relationships (e.g., Adams & Glasner, 1954; Silverman & Powers, 1970; Von Misch, 1952; Salfield, Lord & Dusseldorf, 1950), others suggest that the root of the psychopathology is in the anal stage (e.g., Browne et al., 1963; Pustrom & Speers, 1964). As described in more detail in Chapter 2, the psychodynamic view is not very useful in elucidating specific treatment programs, because mute behavior is considered to be a function of intrapsychic conflicts that are relatively uninfluenced by environmental events.

Although there have been problems in the account of underlying causes of selective mutism, psychodynamic writers have described the ''symptom'' to some degree. In some reports, relatively specific criteria were provided to define parameters of the behavior. For example, Silverman and Powers (1970) used the following criteria to define their subject pool: (1) The children would speak only to the immediate family and close friends and would not speak to strangers or in school; (2) the symptom (we would subsubstitute the term *behavior*) was not a transitory one and had to exist for a period of at least 2 years; (3) the symptom would not yield to the usual interventions one would use to engage the child in speech; (4) no severe underlying psychopathology or demonstrable organic disorder could be present; and (5) the children must be functioning in the average range of intelligence [p. 183]. These criteria are relatively stringent when compared to other work in the psychodynamic area. Nevertheless, these criteria generally ignore the role of environmental influences and present many problems in creating an operational definition.

*The Behavior Therapy Model.*    In contrast to the psychodynamic approach, the behavior therapy orientation has perceived mute behavior as a function of antecedent and consequent environmental events that vary across situations, people, and time. The behavior therapy applications in the selective mutism area have more commonly been affiliated with the more strict operant approach as represented in applied behavior analysis (see Kazdin,1978a ,for a discussion of the scope of behavior modification). The behavior therapy approach has different implications for definition of the problem behavior. The particular frequency, intensity, duration, and appropriateness become important in defining a behavior or providing a behavioral diagnosis (cf. Kanfer & Saslow, 1969).

In concert with this view, researchers operating from the behavioral orientation have typically defined mutism in terms of speech in certain situations or under certain stimulus conditions. Yet there remains some definitional problems in the behavior therapy literature (Kratochwill et al., 1979). First, a number of different subjects have been subsumed under the umbrella term *mutism*. For example, although the vast majority of subjects are labeled "electively" or "selectively mute," some subjects have limited functional speech in all situations (e.g., Blake & Moss, 1967). Therefore, their speech is not select with respect to stimulus situations.

Another issue relates to the frequency of speech in numerous situations. Some writers have included a low frequency of speech across all situations in the selective mutism category (e.g., Calhoun & Koenig, 1973). Yet this deviates considerably from the literature that identifies this as a problem of no speech in certain stimulus situations. This is not a problem insofar as developing an effective treatment strategy, because presumably, the same procedures used for low-frequency speech could be used for zero-frequency speech (see also the Chapter 7 discussion regarding this issue). However, related to this is a problem of terminology that may obscure research in the area. Although many behavior therapists employ conventional diagnostic terms to facilitate communication (e.g., phobias, schizophrenia, and so forth), the development of new terms to distinguish selective mutism from other patterns seems to be misplaced precision. For example, the suggestion by Williamson et al. (1977b) to use the term *reluctant speech* to refer to *low* frequency of speech in some settings may serve to obscure the major goal of behavioral assessment—that is, a specific operational assessment of the target behavior by direct means.

*Recommendations.*    The term *selective mutism* covers the vast majority of cases reviewed in this book. The major goal of definition should be a careful assessment of the behavior, so that the lack of verbal behavior can be defined in terms of frequency, intensity, duration, and social appropriateness. The advantages of this approach have already been elucidated in other sections and chapters. Suffice it to say that the researchers should gather data on the frequency, intensity, duration, and appropriateness of speech across a number of different stimulus situations (e.g., home, school, individuals, and so on). The mutism could then be defined as the lack of speech over different stimulus situations. The advantages of this lie in the avoidance of constructs (typical in the psychodynamic model), the avoidance of debates over terminology (*elective, selective, reluctant,* and so forth), and the conceptualization of treatment programs and procedures to facilitate maintenance and generalization of behavior changes. Thus, in this context, treatment procedures from a variety of areas of children's disorders could be employed.

## Scope of Therapeutic Focus

Selective mutism rarely occurs as the only problem behavior the child is displaying. Most writers have noted that such children also evidence avoidance and social withdrawal behaviors. Some children may not attend school, whereas others have poor academic and social skills. Thus, it must be strongly emphasized that in addition to assessment of the selective mutism, the researcher must focus attention on aspects of the child's behavior that may also cause current and future adjustment problems. Indeed, a careful analysis of the child's behavior may demonstrate that the selective mutism is but one of several primary difficulties. Moreover, the family may be in need of psychotherapeutic services because of any number of serious problems in the home.

   Selective mutism has sometimes been included as a behavior that is part of a more pervasive pattern of anxiety or avoidance behaviors (cf. Richards & Siegel, 1978, for an overview). Richards and Siegel (1978) noted that clinicians who do not recognize, assess, and directly intervene with the withdrawn child's social skill deficits are unlikely to be successful (see also Gelfand, 1979). Moreover, socially isolated children frequently have socially awkward parents (cf. Sherman & Farina, 1974), suggesting that the entire family may profit from social skill training.

Social withdrawal or isolation has received increased attention in the research literature (Amidon, 1961; Amidon & Hoffman, 1975; Asher, Oden, & Gottman, 1977; Bonney, 1971; Brison, 1966; Guerney & Flumen, 1970; Hops, Walker, & Greenwood, 1977; Strain, Cooke, & Apolloni, 1976). Social skill training programs have also been designed for such children (Hops et al., 1977; O'Connor, 1969, 1972). One issue that then arises in treatment of selective mutism is that there may be a number of co-occurring behaviors that need assessment and therapeutic intervention. Hôw might these behaviors be identified, assessed, and subsequently treated? One way to conceptualize this area is to examine the child's behaviors in terms of *deficits*. Doke (1976) provided the following conceptualization of deficit behavior:

A child may be said to have a deficit if he lacks a skill that is required in daily living, socialization, or task performance. Or, a child may be described as having a behavioral deficit. Furthermore, the term "deficit" need not only apply to behaviors that are unlearned. It may also apply to behaviors that have been learned, but are not exhibited well enough or frequently enough (i.e., low-probability behaviors) [p. 495].

Within this conceptualization, the researcher/clinician can use the general methods of behavioral assessment to design a treatment program on dimensions of behavioral deficits.

Another lead to assessment of co-occurring behaviors comes from the pattern of behaviors that Quay (1979) has identified as "anxiety withdrawal." Quay (1979) has described some frequently found characteristics that define this pattern of behavior (see Table 6.3). Children within the "anxiety-withdrawal" category have deficit-type behaviors. Generally, the behaviors identified in Table 6.3 by Quay (1979) are overt and therefore subject to direct methods of be-

TABLE 6.3
Some Characteristics Defining Anxiety Withdrawal[a]

1. Anxious, fearful, tense
2. Shy, timid, bashful
3. Withdrawn, seclusive, friendless
4. Depressed, sad, disturbed
5. Hypersensitive, easily hurt
6. Self-conscious, easily embarrassed
7. Feels inferior, worthless
8. Lacks self-confidence
9. Easily flustered
10. Aloof
11. Cries frequently
12. Reticent, secretive

[a]After Quay (1979, p. 18).

havioral assessment. However, some characteristics are more inferential (e.g., self-conscious, inferiority feelings), and therefore it may be difficult to obtain reliable and valid measures on them.

## Research Design

Many therapeutic research strategies in the psychotherapy literature use group or multiunit designs. The primary research strategy in the mutism literature has involved intensive study of the single case. This is typical in the study of many rare behavior disorders such as specific phobias. A major methodological concern in the selective mutism literature is whether the observed behavior would have occurred without the experimental (therapeutic) manipulations. This issue gains special significance when one considers that many of the therapeutic programs were implemented over months or even years. One could expect maturational or social changes to produce changes in children, so any research must be carefully designed to isolate the therapeutic variables responsible for change and rule out time-related changes.

An examination of Table 6.1 and Table 6.2 presents a somewhat discouraging picture when experimental design is considered. Table 6.1 shows that all therapeutic reports in the psychodynamic literature involved case study methodology, a procedure characterized by no formal data, subjective interpretation of changes, and no design to assist in experimental analysis. The case study procedure has been characteristic of much psychotherapy research for the past 50 years and has severely curtailed its credibility (cf. Hersen & Barlow, 1976).

An examination of the behavior therapy research presented in Table 6.2 also suggests that many authors have used case study methodology (approximately 50%). Many authors in the behavior therapy literature used more formal measurement strategies (e.g., Norman & Broman, 1970) and/or basic AB designs (e.g., Blake & Moss, 1967; Nash et al., 1979; Williamson et al., 1977a), but these strategies also have severe methodological weaknesses (cf. Hersen & Barlow, 1976; Kratochwill, 1978, 1979). Very few studies employed design and assessment criteria that allowed an analysis of therapeutic mechanisms (e.g., Griffith et al., 1975; Munford et al., 1976; Piersel & Kratochwill, in press; Sanok & Striefel, 1979; Wulbert et al., 1973). Unfortunately, in the Munford et al. (1976) study, concomitant psychotherapy makes interpretations of the outcome difficult.

*Case Study Methodology.* The case study method severely limits statements that can be made regarding therapeutic outcomes. A major problem in the psychodynamic literature with case study methodology is the subjective nature of interpretations made about the intervention program and outcomes. This is related to the model that emphasizes underlying personality dynamics to explain behavior change. Nevertheless, single-subject research in this area does not have to be limited to case study methodology. Two methodologists affiliated with psychodynamic therapy have gone beyond the complete subjective representation of data and have begun to construct a more adequate technology for single-case research (cf. Chassan, 1967; Shapiro, 1961, 1966), but selective mutism research has remained uninfluenced by their work. An important contribution of Shapiro was the utilization of carefully constructed measures of clinically relevant responses administered repeatedly over time in a single case. For example, Shapiro examined fluctuations in these measures and hypothesized controlling effects of therapeutic variables. However, many of these studies were correlational, a procedure Shapiro (1966) referred to as simple or complex descriptive studies. Chassan (1967) also illustrated the uses of single-case designs in psychotherapy research, particularly psychoanalysis. Chassan concentrated on correlational-type designs using trend analysis, but some procedures involved prototypes of the ABA design, which extended Shapiro's work but contained some of the same methodological flaws (cf. Hersen & Barlow, 1976).

Some behavioral researchers have stressed that despite limitations, the case study method can make a contribution to experimental effort (e.g., Kratochwill, 1978; Lazarus & Davidson, 1971). In this review of single-case designs, Hersen and Barlow (1976) summarized some contributions by suggesting that case study methodology can: (1) foster clinical innovation; (2) cast doubt on certain theoretical assumptions; (3) permit study of rare phenomena; (4) develop new technical skills; (5) buttress theoretical views; (6) promote refinement in technique; and (7) provide clinical data that can be used to design more highly controlled research. Presumably, case study research can generate hypotheses for subsequent research (cf. Bolgar, 1965; Lazarus & Davidson, 1971), as has been true in the selective mutism literature. However, case study research can involve "misplaced precision," for a researcher's efforts would be better spent on a more well controlled experiment wherein appropriate design and assessment criteria are employed (cf. Kratochwill, 1978). Case study research is subject to all major sources of threats to internal and external validity, and it would be better to use a more credible methodology where possible. This is especially true in the mutism literature, where a large number of case studies already exist, making the need to move forward with more credible methodology apparent.

*Basic or AB Designs.*    Several authors conducting research on the disorder of selective mutism employed a basic or AB design (e.g., Blake & Moss, 1967; Calhoun & Koenig, 1973; Nash et al., 1979; Straughan et al., 1965). In this research strategy, which occurred in the behavior therapy literature, repeated direct measurement of a target behavior (speaking) was gathered over time to establish first a baseline measure. After stability was achieved, an intervention was introduced, and changes in the target behavior were noted. This design differs from the aforementioned case study methodology in that a baseline is taken and the intervention is compared against this baseline series. This AB design represents an improved form of the pretest–posttest design (see Campbell & Stanley, 1966) in that more frequent measurement is taken, reducing (but *not eliminating*) some invalidity threats (cf. Kratochwill, 1978). Hersen and Barlow (1976) noted that the AB design has been useful in psychotherapeutic research with: (1) a single target measure and extended follow-up; (2) multiple target measures; and (3) follow-up and booster treatments. Unfortunately, the AB design limitations outweigh its potential advantages. First, researchers using the AB designs are unable to rule out historical and many other time-related confounds. Another problem is that there is difficulty in interpreting an intervention effect with baseline trend. When the baseline series is stable or is in the opposite direction from the expected treatment, or the treatment exhibits a significant shift in the series, interpretation is not as difficult. However, a strong case for the treatment can only be made when the effects are replicated, which requires a more credible design.

*Recommended Design Options.*    Single-case behavior therapy research designs have proliferated in recent years, with advantages and disadvantages of these procedures elucidated in many sources (e.g., Bailey, 1977; Glass, Willson, & Gottman, 1975; Hersen & Barlow, 1976; Kazdin, 1980b; Kratochwill, 1978; Robinson & Foster, 1979; Thoresen, in press). Although a large number of experiments conducted in behavior therapy involved one subject, designs in this area are not limited to one subject (e.g., in the Calhoun and Koenig (1973) study, a group composed the experimental unit). Single-case designs have been extensively developed and employed in behavior therapy, but they are not limited to this orientation.

Several unique characteristics of single-case designs can be identified (Hersen & Barlow, 1976; Kazdin & Wilson, 1978; Kratochwill, 1978, 1979). Single-case designs generally promote the observation of overt behavior (direct assessment), continuous assessment of behavior, data-based decisions about treatment, and, recently, specific criteria for assessing the reliability and importance of therapeutic change. It is beyond the scope of this book to detail the various characteristics of these designs, and the reader should consult a number of direct sources (e.g., Hersen & Barlow, 1976; Kratochwill, 1978; Thoresen, in press).

Several limitations of these designs have also been suggested. The major problem relates to the generalization of results from a single subject. A researcher may develop an effective technique for treatment of selective mutism, but there is frequently little basis for inferring that this therapeutic procedure would be equally effective when applied to clients with a similar behavior disorder (i.e., another case of selective mutism; client generality), or that different therapists using the procedure would achieve the same results (therapist generality), or that the technique would work in different settings (setting generality). Although there are answers to this problem in terms of direct, systematic, and clinical replication procedures (cf. Hersen & Barlow, 1976), replication is a long and difficult process and may not easily be attained by one or a group of researchers (cf. Kazdin & Wilson, 1978; Kratochwill, 1979). This is especially a problem in the case of relatively rare disorders such as selective mutism. Finally, criteria for evaluating change, particularly graphical analysis, may prove troublesome unless statistical analysis is employed (see Kratochwill, 1979).

These limitations notwithstanding, and I have by no means listed them all, the single-subject research design appears to be the methodology of choice in research on selective mutism. In this context, the single-case research strategy provides an empirical and scientific basis for evaluating treatment of mute clients, is generally the methodology of choice in mutism research (cf. Kratochwill et al., 1979), allows the building of effective interventions by adding components to enhance therapeutic change in a cumulative fashion (Kazdin & Wilson, 1978), and allows comparison of different treatments with the mute client.

The investigator who designs an intervention program for the mute client should structure the design to demonstrate the specific contribution of the treatment. Although a variety of different single-subject designs can be used, in mutism research, the conventional ABAB intrasubject replication design may typically be inappropriate with respect to the necessity for a treatment withdrawal or reversal and ethical considerations in a return to baseline phase. The reversal variation possibly has more utility (e.g., Munford et al., 1976) than the withdrawal variation because it circumvents a withdrawal of contingencies. As an alternative to the ABAB design, the selective mutism researcher should consider three other possible design options; these include the multiple baseline, the alternating-treatment design, and the changing-criterion design. The alternating-treatment design (Barlow & Hayes, 1979) or "simultaneous treatment" design (Hersen & Barlow, 1976; Kazdin, 1977b; Kazdin & Hartmann, 1978; Kratochwill, 1978) examines the effect of different interventions, each of which is implemented in the same phase of the program.[2] The design appears useful when the investigator is interested in determining which among two or more procedures is more effective. In the design, a baseline observation on a single response is first completed, and then two or more interventions are implemented in the same phase but under varied stimulus conditions. For example, two interventions could be compared by implementing them on a given day in the intervention phase, with one in the morning and the other in the afternoon. The treatments can be varied across periods of the day (e.g., morning and afternoon) and across staff or caretakers (e.g., teachers or parents). The different treatments are balanced across all conditions so that their effects can be separated from these conditions. The treatment phase is continued, varying conditions of administra-

---

[2]The "alternating-treatments design" has been termed, variously, a multielement baseline design, a multiple schedule design, and a randomization design. Barlow and Hayes (1979) have recently reviewed the critical differences between the design and the simultaneous treatment design.

tion, until responses stabilize under separate treatments. The design is not without limitations: (1) A large number of sessions are required so that each treatment can be administered by a given therapist and across time periods an equal number of times; (2) a client may not discriminate different contingencies correlated with a particular treatment; and (3) the effects of administering each treatment in the same phase may differ from what they would be if the treatments were administered in separate phases (cf. Kazdin, 1977b).

Another design that would be especially useful for evaluating treatment effects with selective mutism, particularly where gradual shaping procedures are used as part of the treatment program, is called the changing-criterion design (see Hall & Fox, 1977; Hartmann & Hall, 1976; Kratochwill, 1978). Munford et al. (1976) used an early variation of this design (see Fig. 5.13, Chapter 5). The changing-criterion design requires initial baseline observations on a single target behavior. Subsequent to the baseline, a treatment program is implemented in each of a series of intervention phases. A stepwise change in criterion rate for mutism would be applied during each treatment phase. Thus, each phase of the design can be conceptualized as a baseline for each subsequent phase. Experimental control would be demonstrated through successive replication of change in the target behavior, which should change with each stepwise change in criterion. Criteria changes function analogously to the sequential changes in behavior, situation, or individual to which (or whom) an intervention is applied in variants of the multiple baseline design. Munford et al. (1976) employed an early variant of the changing-criterion design in which the recent methodological refinements (e.g., baseline and systematic criterion shifts) were not specified. The reader is referred to Kratochwill (1978) for a more detailed discussion of the design.

Finally, the multiple baseline design would be especially useful because it has application across responses, situations, and individuals. Its use across situations (settings or time) provides a useful research strategy for selective mutism, because speech appears to be select with respect to situations. For example, baseline data for a given verbal response could be collected across two or more situations or settings, such as the classroom, or the playground, and in other situations where talking does not occur. After behavior has stabilized in each situation, the intervention is applied sequentially to each situation given that stability was achieved in former baselines. The specific effect of the intervention would be shown if talking were to change in a particular situation only when the intervention was introduced. However, in the multiple baseline across situations, an unambiguous demonstration of the intervention depends on changes in behavior only in those situations in which the treatment is in effect. In some cases, changing behavior in one situation has changed behavior in other situations in which the intervention was not introduced (e.g., Bennett & Maley, 1973; Kazdin, 1973b). Thus, although this version of the multiple baseline design may not unambiguously demonstrate a functional relation if situations are so similar that altering behavior in one situation changes behavior in another, generalized effects across different baselines appear to be an exception rather than the rule (cf. Kazdin, 1977b).

The multiple baseline across situations is useful when one mute client can be treated across different settings. In rare instances, two or more mute clients may come to the attention of the therapist at approximately the same time, as in the case of twins (e.g., Mora et al., 1962; Piersel & Kratochwill, in press), or the researcher working in a clinic or school setting may receive two or more selective mutism referrals at approximately the same time. In such instances, the researcher could employ a multiple baseline across subjects. The logic behind the design's application across subjects is the same as in its use across settings or time. It is generally recognized that at least three or, if possible, four subjects should be included to increase inference for a functional relation. However, the selective mutism researcher working with three or two subjects could combine the multiple baseline design with another procedure (such as the changing-criterion design) to increase experimental credibility. As is true in the multiple baseline's application across situations or time, experimental units (i.e., subjects) should remain as independent as possible. An example of the application of the multiple baseline design in the selective mutism literature occurs in the Piersel and Kratochwill (in press) report, where a combination across-subjects and -settings design was employed (see Fig. 5.23 in Chapter 5), and in the Griffith et al. (1975) study, where a treatment was administered across settings (see Fig. 5.24 in Chapter 5).

## Systematic Treatment Evaluation Strategies

An examination of Table 6.2 demonstrates that a variety of behavioral treatment procedures were employed in the treatment of selective mutism, with the application of straightforward reinforcement (typically social and tangible) being used most frequently. Many cases of selective mutism have been treated with stimulus-fading procedures (e.g., Conrad et al., 1974; Wulbert et al., 1973), shaping procedures (e.g., Blake & Moss, 1967), aversive control procedures (Shaw, 1971; Van der Kooy & Webster, 1975), or contingency management (e.g., Piersel & Kratochwill, in press; Williamson et al., 1977b). More commonly, authors used a number of therapeutic procedures simultaneously without analysis of separate components. Yet some procedures just mentioned may be effective when combined with other treatment procedures. For example, Wulbert et al. (1973) found that stimulus fading was a necessary component of the treatment process. Whereas the time-out contingency was found to facilitate treatment if combined with stimulus fading, it was completely ineffective without the stimulus fading. Findings like these raise the issue of which therapeutic procedure, singly or in combination, is the most desirable to implement in the treatment of selective mutism. Generally, there has been little systematic attempt in the behavior therapy treatment of selective mutism to tease apart the relative contribution of various treatment strategies or to prescribe the best method of therapeutic applications. Presumably, one major reason for this is that no adequate technology has been available for this endeavor.

In recent years, there has been increasing recognition that comparison of different therapeutic techniques in applied settings is important (cf. Hersen & Barlow, 1976; Kazdin & Wilson, 1978). However, comparing different treatments without an adequate assessment of other research issues can impede as well as promote progress in the development of effective therapeutic techniques (Kazdin & Wilson, 1978). For example, although some selective mutism researchers described various components of the therapeutic manipulations, rarely were the operative processes systematically monitored. Also, a large number of studies (both psychodynamic and behavioral) involved the client in concomitant therapies during the manipulation of the major therapeutic variable. Thus, even with a credible research design, the additional therapeutic involvement makes suspect the conclusion that behavior change was due to the major therapeutic variable.

Different therapeutic evaluation strategies have recently been suggested (cf. Kazdin, 1979; Kazdin & Wilson, 1978). These include the treatment package, constructive, dismantling, parametric, comparative, client–therapist variation, and internal structure or process strategies. It is beyond the scope of this chapter to detail these strategies and the issues accompanying their use, so only some highlights are presented (see Kazdin, 1979, for an overview).

The treatment package strategy refers to evaluation of the effects of a given treatment as that treatment is typically implemented or advocated by proponents of the technique. The package typically includes several components. In the constructive treatment strategy, a treatment is developed by adding components to enhance therapy-effects technique. In the dismantling strategy, research is aimed at understanding the basis for behavior change effected by the overall package and begins to analyze the influence of specific components. The parametric treatment strategy refers to varying specific aspects of the treatment to determine how to maximize change; it bears similarity to the constructive strategy insofar as its purpose is to examine dimensions that can be used to enhance therapeutic effects. Comparison strategies involve direct comparison of different treatments. The client-and-therapist variation strategy examines these components by initially selecting clients and therapists for specific attributes or, alternatively, by experimentally manipulating the behavior of clients or therapists. Finally, internal structure or process strategies examine the change over the process of therapy and so represent one dimension of the conventional notion of outcome.

Many of these treatment/research strategies are conducted in the context of multiunit or comparative group studies, but single-case methodology does allow the building of effective treatments by either adding or withdrawing components to enhance therapeutic change in a cumulative fashion (Kazdin, 1978). For example, "interaction"-type designs discussed by Hersen and Barlow (1976) or multiunit ($N = 1$) interaction designs reviewed by Kratochwill (1978) can be employed if enough subjects are available.

With regard to the selective mutism literature, research has generally followed no specific strategy in refining therapeutic techniques. The adoption of any particular strategy will likely depend on the extent to which certain procedures are investigated.

Of course, the use of various treatment strategies depends greatly on the use of a credible methodology to investigate singly effective techniques. Because research on selective mutism is quite primitive with respect to methodology, the more fundamental issue is to assess therapeutic variables critically with credible research strategies in the future. Kratochwill et al. (1979) made the recommendations for future work in the selective mutism area (see also Callner, 1975, for similar suggestions in the research on drug abuse). First, researchers should be encouraged (typically through publications) to report *controlled* intervention studies whether the treatment was successful or unsuccessful. It may be more important to isolate and discuss the conditions surrounding an ineffective treatment in the context of a well-controlled study than to demonstrate "success" in a poorly controlled study (i.e., like a large number of reported studies in the selective mutism literature). Second, replication research appears essential in the selective mutism area. Systematic, direct, and clinical replication procedures should be considered wherever possible (see Hersen & Barlow, 1976). Few researchers in the selective mutism area have extended their own work (see, however, Williamson et al., 1977a, 1977b). Finally, researchers should appraise their studies on variables similar to those presented in Tables 6.1 and 6.2. These variables, as well as the factors elucidated in this chapter, may provide a list of minimum standards to include and discuss in future research.

## Direct Assessment

In the beginning of this chapter, a case was made for *direct* assessment of behavior as an appropriate method for evaluation of treatment programs for selective mutism. In most cases, but not all of them (see Chapter 4), direct assessment of the target behavior is made through observation in the natural environment. Use of this form of assessment, though preferred in research, presents a number of methodological issues (cf. Gelfand & Hartmann, 1975; Johnson & Bolstad, 1973; Kazdin, 1977b; Kent & Foster, 1977; Wildman & Erickson, 1978). When naturalistic observation is employed, the researcher must attend to observer variables (e.g., training, reactivity, drift, bias), instrumentation variables (e.g., codes, sampling procedures, observer agreement or reliability, training devices), and subject variables, such as the representativeness of the behavior. The vast majority of behavior therapy reports did not address these issues. For example, although observer agreement has been given a great deal of attention in the applied behavioral literature (e.g., Baer, 1977; Hersen & Barlow, 1976; Kazdin, 1977a; Kratochwill & Wetzel, 1977), only 32% of the behavior therapy reports presented reliability data. Of those that did, it is impossible to determine if it was assessed correctly and if various sources of artifact and bias, as well as the characteristics of the assessment itself, contaminated the direct assessment data. Various features of the problem include reactivity of the reliability assessment, observer drift, method of calculating agreement, complexity of response codes and behavioral observations, and observer expectancies and feedback, among others (Kazdin, 1977a). Although future selective mutism research must focus on these factors, they represent only some of the issues that may influence the interpretation of reliability. Indeed, observer agreement and accuracy can be viewed as target behaviors in their own right that are a function of such factors as the observational system; characteristics of the experimenter, observer, client; methods of scoring behavior; the nature and duration of observer training; situational and instructional variables during assessment of reliability; the pattern of client behavior; and concurrent observation of stimulus and consequent events (cf. Kazdin, 1977a).

*Recommendations.* Direct assessment of behavior through naturalistic observation has become increasingly complex, as reflected in the current number of issues known to affect the outcomes when these techniques are used. Again, it is impossible to review all the issues that can facilitate accurate and reliable recording of behavior. Nevertheless, the available literature does provide a number of useful recommendations for use in direct observational assessment (cf. Kent & Foster, 1977; Wildman & Erickson, 1978).

Observer training should include samples of behavioral sequences and environmental settings that closely resemble the behaviors and settings in which data collection will occur. All observers should be trained together and the ratings compared with a single formal criterion. Training must be long enough to ensure that there is agreement to a specified criterion on each code. Various devices such as video- and audiotapes may be used in the training.

Once the research begins, the conditions for assessing observer agreement should be maintained to assure consistent levels of agreement. Wildman and Erickson (1978) noted that continuous overt monitoring and randomized, covert monitoring generate the most stable levels of agreement. Where possible, videotaped sessions may be presented to observers in random order, and training can be continued by having observers match their ratings to a standardized tape.

Observer bias can be reduced by not communicating the specific research hypotheses to experimenters and observers. Possibly, explicit instructions to the observer indicating that the specific outcomes are unknown may be preferable to avoidance of the topic.

In research on selective mutism, specific observational codes must be constructed so that behaviors may be easily rated. Generally, a researcher should be somewhat conservative in the number of codes that are to be rated at any one time. Operational definitions should be tested to ensure that observer agreement estimates are high.

Finally, every attempt should be made to conduct the observations in as unobtrusive a fashion as is possible. In clinic settings, one-way mirrors may be available, but more typically, observers will have to avoid influencing the subjects in natural settings. Data should be closely monitored for any evidence of reactivity or bias.

In the area of observer agreement, the complexity of issues has prompted interest in the use of generalizability theory (cf. Cronbach, Glaser, Nada, Rajaratman, 1972) to conceptualize behavior observations (cf. Coates & Thoresen, 1978; Cone, 1977, 1978; Jones, Reid, & Patterson, 1975; Kazdin, 1977a; Mash & McElwee, 1974; Strossen, Coates, & Thoresen, 1979). Generalizability theory allows conceptualization of reliability for assessment across different conditions within an experiment. For example, it provides a comprehensive method for assessing simultaneously the independent and interactive effects of several factors on an observed score, and it can assist the investigator in the design of assessment procedures so that information-gathering efforts can be distributed to yield as much accuracy as possible (cf. Coates & Thoresen, 1978a). Within this conceptualization, the extent to which observations in a study vary across certain dimensions, such as observers and occasions, can be examined, and the generalizability of the data across different levels of these facets can be evaluated directly. Despite some controversy over its application (cf. Jones, 1978), future researchers on selective mutism should consider that an advantage of generalizability theory is that it simultaneously examines the contribution of diverse characteristics of data assessment.

## Outcome Evaluation Criteria

In this book, a case has been made for the direct assessment of behavior as opposed to indirect measurement systems such as subjective reports or personality tests. Recently, broader criteria have been proposed for evaluation of therapy (cf. Kazdin, 1978b, 1979; Kazdin & Wilson, 1978). The criteria discussed in this section include the criteria for evaluation (visual and/or statistical), social validation, breadth of changes, durability of therapeutic change, and efficiency and cost-related criteria.

*Criteria for Evaluation.*    When data have been collected and an appropriate design is used to control major sources of invalidity, the issue of an appropriate method of data analysis arises. The application of various analytic methods in a single-subject experiment complements the design to assist in drawing conclusions from the data and therefore constitutes an important validity issue (Kratochwill, 1979). In the behavior therapy reports using single-subject designs, the data analytic method consisted of visual analysis of the graphical data plot. However, this analytic procedure may not always be appropriate.

In recent years there has been increasing controversy over whether visual *or* statistical analytic methods should be employed (see Kazdin, 1976; Kratochwill, 1978, 1979; for an overview). The former consists of a procedure in which the researcher plots the experimental data wherein the plot represents a graphic pattern corresponding to various design phases. A judgment of the effect is made regarding the outcome. The statistical procedure is characterized by the application of an inferential test wherein a decision rule based on probability estimates is made.

It is no secret that there has been a raging controversy over the application of statistical tests in applied behavioral research. Suffice it to say that the issues are complex, but the ''either/or'' flavor of the debate has not been resolved. Recently, visual analysis has been considerably refined and formal guidelines established for its use (see Parsonson & Baer, 1978). The advances made in this area should promote better use of graphical analysis, but a major limitation of these procedures remains—namely, the unreliable nature of this analysis tactic (cf. Kratochwill & Levin, 1979), particularly with autocorrelated data.[3]

A vareity of statistical procedures have been advocated, but those techniques that fail to account for the correlated error in time-series data (e.g., ANOVA, regression) are inappropriate (cf. Kratochwill, 1978; Levin, Marascuilo, & Hubert, 1978). Appropriate procedures include time-series analysis (Glass et al., 1975; Gottman & Glass, 1978) and nonparametric randomization tests (Edgington, 1967; Levin et al., 1978). The nonparametric approaches are noted for their simplicity, whereas the time-series analyses are more rigorous and mathematically formidable. The future will likely see an increase in the use of statistical procedures in single-case research.

## Social Validation

Recent work in applied behavior analysis suggests that experimental and therapeutic criteria be employed in therapeutic research (cf. Kazdin, 1977b; Kazdin & Wilson, 1978; Risley, 1970; Wolf, 1978). The experimental criterion

---

[3]Autocorrelation refers to a correlation ($r$) between data points separated by different time intervals (or lags) in time-series data. An autocorrelation of the first lag is computed by pairing the initial observation with the second, second with the third, third with the fourth, and so forth throughout the series (see Gottman & Leiblum, 1974; Kazdin, 1976). Use of various statistical tests (e.g., ANOVA and regression procedures) requires that the *errors* in the statistical model are uncorrelated (i.e., ''independent'' if the normality assumption holds). Errors (or *residuals*) refer to what is left of an observation after it has been deviated about the model's parameters (e.g., a grand mean, treatment effects; see Levin et al., 1978).

involves comparison of the target behavior before and after the intervention has been applied. The aforementioned discussion of visual and statistical analysis relates to criteria for the experimental criterion. In addition to experimental criteria, researchers should be concerned with therapeutic or clinical criteria for behavior change, a procedure that has been referred to as social validation (cf. Kazdin, 1977b; see also discussion in Chapter 1). Selection of certain criteria presupposes that behavior selected for therapeutic involvement is itself of social significance (i.e., elimination of selective mutism). Achieving therapeutic change of social significance also presupposes a criterion toward which therapeutic strategies can develop and against which program outcomes can be evaluated. When evaluating a treatment outcome, two social validation procedures are involved. First, the behavior of the client is compared to that of his or her peers who have not been identified as problematic. In selective mutism research, normal-speaking peers would be observed to establish a criterion level. Second, subjective evaluations of the subject's target behavior by individuals in the natural environment are solicited. Thus, therapeutic changes can be viewed as clinically important if the intervention has brought the client's performance within the range of socially acceptable levels, as evidenced by the child's peer group, or if the client's behavior is judged by others as reflecting a qualitative improvement on global ratings (Kazdin, 1977b).

Formalized measures of social validation have only recently been reported in the literature (see Kazdin, 1977b; Maloney, Harper, Braukmann, Fixsen, Phillips, & Wolf, 1976; for examples). Although no researchers in the selective mutism area employed social validation in a formalized fashion, many did interview teachers, parents, and other socialization agents to establish some external validation criterion (e.g., Piersel & Kratochwill, in press). In future research efforts, these procedures should become more formalized. It should be noted that social validation of outcomes should enter into an acceptable range when judged by socialization agents. It is doubtful that the establishment of minimal verbal behavior in a few isolated situations or with the therapist will be socially significant. Therapeutic or clinical outcomes should far surpass experimental criteria in the research design, visual and/or statistical criteria notwithstanding.

*Breadth of Changes.*    A related concern on outcome measures relates to the breadth of therapeutic change. Presumably, researchers could meet therapeutic criteria through change in the verbal behavior of the client (i.e., the problem for which "the client or his/her parent, teacher or legal guardian sought" treatment). Another criterion that can be invoked to validate treatment is the breadth of change produced that relates to an extension of therapeutic effects beyond the target problem (Kazdin & Wilson, 1978). For example, through increased verbal behavior, one might expect that other social and academic behaviors would improve. Though this has been mentioned by most selective mutism researchers, such measures could be made more formal.

Equally important to consider would be any negative or adverse effects that are produced by the treatment, particularly when aversive procedures are employed. In addition to meeting ethical obligations (see Chapter 7), formal measurement of such side effects would allow prompt intervention when necessary. Kazdin and Wilson (1978) noted:

> Generally, the breadth and nature of changes are important criteria for evaluating a given treatment or for comparing the relative utility of different treatments. Presumably, different treatments develop different skills in clients and are likely to vary in the generality of effects produced. While the primary criterion for change necessarily is improvement in the problem for which treatment is sought, the nature and extent of changes beyond this focus also are important [pp. 120–121].

*Durability of Changes.*   The importance of maintenance of therapeutic changes as well as generalization of change has been stressed in this chapter (see pp. 134–136). The durability of change should also be considered as an outcome evaluation criterion. This issue is especially important when considering that two procedures that result in equal therapeutic change on outcome may have differential effects or follow-up. Suggestions presented earlier should be considered for assessment of the durability of change.

*Efficiency and Cost-Related Criteria.*   In addition to the foregoing criteria, future selective mutism researchers should consider criteria related to the efficiency in duration of therapy, efficiency in the manner of administering the treatment, client costs, and cost-effectiveness (cf. Kazdin & Wilson, 1978). Efficiency in duration of therapy implies that a procedure that reaches a specified level of improvement in a shorter period of time is preferred (keeping in mind the other criteria already discussed, such as durability of change). In the mutism literature, psychodynamic studies extended over months and even years. Generally, the behavior therapy procedures were considerably shorter and usually had much better results on outcome, generalization, and follow-up (see also Kratochwill et al., 1979). Within behavior therapy, different procedures may yield the same results but save considerable time. Williamson et al. (1977b) noted that elaborate procedures such as stimulus fading, shaping, or aversive procedures were probably much more time-consuming than their contingency management program where some speech was already evident. Thus, accurate assessment should presumably save time in the long run. And, time-efficiency can also be compared against the severity of the problem. Many of the children referred for treatment were mute for extensive periods of time. Rasbury (1974) noted that "even though we felt the therapeutic procedure might have been altered to facilitate quicker behavioral change, the total amount of time invested in daily sessions (23 hours for 140 sessions) was remarkably short in contrast with the six-year duration of selective mutism exhibited by this child [p. 104]."

Efficiency can also be measured through the manner in which the treatment program is administered. Piersel and Kratochwill (in press) noted that their consultation services (cf. Bergan, 1977)[4] were time-efficient relative to other procedures that might have been employed. When a teacher administers the program in the classroom, this should be more efficient than if the behavior therapist becomes directly involved. Many behavior therapy reports note the use of paraprofessionals and natural socialization agents, such as teachers (e.g., Conrad et al., 1974; Dmitriev & Hawkins, 1973; Rasbury, 1974). Such procedures may also assist in durability and generalization (Stokes & Baer, 1977) and so should be considered in outcome efficiency measures.

Client costs should also be examined in the therapeutic program. Costs can be either monetary or "emotional." In the case of monetary expense, client costs are influenced by such factors as the cost of professional training of the therapist and the disseminability of treatment (Kazdin & Wilson, 1978). Future research should consider the treatment setting (clinic vs. school), therapist (behavior therapist vs. teacher or paraprofessional), and the cost-effectiveness of the treatment itself (reinforcement vs. time-out). Based upon estimates of the cost of treatment for the treatment of the two cases of selective mutism, Williamson et al. (1977b) noted that through proper client assessment of some speech (what they label as "reluctant speech") and the use of a less time-consuming procedure (contingency management as compared to reinforcement sampling, escape, and so forth; see pp. 93–99), a saving of from $240 to $330 per case was made. Thus, accurate assessment can be important for therapy as well as for cost-effectiveness.

## SUMMARY AND CONCLUSIONS

An increasing concern with therapeutic efforts in the research on selective mutism must include the various methodological and conceptual issues that accompany both psychodynamic and behavior therapy research. In this chapter I discussed the importance of specific outcome measures. Generalization must be both assessed and programmed, and this is true of follow-up (maintenance) measures as well. More specific operational definitions of selective mutism must be provided, with less reliance on inferential measures. Behaviors that co-occur with selective mutism must also be assessed and targeted for intervention, given that they are problematic. Direct assessment of these behaviors seems most important in future work in this area, as well as the use of systematic evaluation and design strategies. Some examples of procedures helpful in this regard were provided. Finally, on outcome evaluation criteria, attention to such components as criteria for evaluation, social validation, breadth of changes, and efficiency and cost-related criteria was emphasized for future research efforts.

---

[4]The behavioral consultation program is based on a model developed by Bergan (1977) and consists of four stages: problem identification, problem analysis, plan intervention, and plan evaluation. The model is most typically implemented through a series of interviews wherein a consultant (e.g., a psychologist) meets with a consultee (e.g., a teacher, a parent).

# 7

## Recommendations for Treatment

This chapter focuses on issues and procedures that are involved in altering selective mutism. The emphasis is primarily on applied behavior analysis procedures in the operant tradition. My emphasis on more operant approaches should not be construed as an overall endorsement of only the operant approach for the treatment of all childhood problems or even for the treatment of selective mutism. Other procedures, such as systematic desensitization, have been successful in the treatment of selective mutism and are discussed later. Nevertheless, the vast majority of behavior therapy research reports employed operant-based techniques, many of which appeared quite effective with mute children. As noted in previous chapters, an important consideration in research and therapy involves application of procedures that facilitate maintenance and generalization. A number of procedures known to facilitate these factors are reviewed. Finally, ethical considerations are discussed in the context of treatment of selective mutism. Before describing some of the therapeutic procedures themselves, I briefly present a perspective on research and practice.

## SOME PERSPECTIVES ON RESEARCH AND PRACTICE

In Chapter 6, a variety of methodological issues were reviewed. Procedures were suggested for analysis of specific techniques in applied single-subject research. Many individuals working in applied settings have the opportunity and the interest in conducting research, so many of these procedures can serve as guidelines. However, many practitioners have a commitment to discovering a treatment that ameliorates a specific behavior problem, rather than adhering to principles of applied research (e.g., credible designs, reliability, and so forth).

A number of authors have suggested that single-case experimental designs are useful to the practitioner in evaluating applied interventions (e.g., Hersen & Barlow, 1976; Kratochwill & Bergan, 1978; Leitenberg, 1973). For example, Hersen and Barlow (1976) noted that one of the major advantages of single-case designs is that this approach "tends to merge the role of scientist-practitioner [p. 356]." Kratochwill and Bergan (1978) noted that although direct service through behavioral consultation does not typically involve a strict research methodology (e.g., economy of effort is promoted through application of procedures that maximize behavior change), applied behavioral research gives the scientist-practitioner model the clearest formulation for *developing* competencies important for the professional psychologist.

Critics of this position (cf. Franks & Wilson, 1977; Kazdin & Wilson, 1978) suggest that there is only a superficial resemblance between single-case design and clinical practice; namely, unlike multiunit research, single-subject research addresses the individual, who is also the practicing therapist's concern. There are several issues raised that may militate against this formulation of the scientist-practitioner role. First, the ethical, practical, and methodological problems inherent in single-case designs are not significantly fewer than conventional multiunit designs. This appears to have increasing validity because of the evolving sophistication of single-case research in terms of design and methodology (cf. Kratochwill, 1978). Second, it is argued that clinically relevant change in the fastest and least expensive means possible is a goal of clinical practice (cf. Azrin, 1977). Package programs may be employed where determining the specific influence of isolated variables must yield to rapid therapeutic change. Third, according to some writers (e.g., Franks & Wilson, 1977), there is little evidence for practitioners employing single-case experimental designs. Moreover, the plea for analysis of psychotherapy strategies outside the behavior therapy orientation to be evaluated by single-case designs (Bergin & Strupp, 1970; Kratochwill, 1979) has not generally been answered. Although Franks and Wilson (1977) presented no data to substantiate this claim, there is evidence that even behavioral practitioners find behavior assessment devices difficult to use and frequently fall back on conventional testing practices (cf. Wade & Baker, 1977, discussed in Chapter 2). Finally, applied clinical research using single-subject designs and their corresponding replication procedures has been employed by skilled, research-oriented investigators (e.g., Hersen & Barlow, 1976) working in settings that support research activities. Likely, individuals working in settings where such reinforcement does not occur would not indulge in large amounts of research.

These issues stand as impressive arguments against the stance that single-subject research blends the scientist-practitioner model. Although one can generally agree with these points, an alternative consideration should be pointed out. Practitioners appropriately trained in applied single-case research methodology have the *potential* to do such research. Many work in settings where research is possible (e.g., schools; cf. Kratochwill, 1977; Kratochwill & Bergan, 1978), and many do conduct research from time to time, even though they are unable to perform the extensive replication procedures advocated by Hersen and Barlow (1976). Moreover, training in applied research methodology has application beyond the conduct of research per se. Particularly for practitioners, it provides a perspective from which to *evaluate* published applied research studies—the source of many psychotherapeutic techniques.

## TREATMENT APPLICATIONS

The analysis of therapeutic procedures for the treatment of selective mutism has been analyzed across both psychodynamic and behavior therapy approaches. The analysis of these two contrasting approaches to treatment suggests that the behavior therapy methods are at least as effective as, and in most cases more effective than, the psychodynamic approaches, methodological limitations notwithstanding. This author believes that behavior therapy remains the treatment of choice with selective mutism. This conclusion is generally consistent with comparative outcome research reviewed by Kazdin and Wilson (1978) in a broader context. These authors note:

> The belief that traditional psychotherapy enjoys data-based empirical support against which behavior therapy has somehow to prove itself has assumed the status of a de facto truth. There might be reasons for preferring traditional psychotherapy over behavior therapy, but the notion that empirical considerations provide a justification is pure fiction [p. 177].

### Behavior Therapy Treatment Approaches

Widespread application of behavior modification approaches has occurred rapidly in the past few years and extends over a large number of different problems and settings (cf. Kazdin, 1978a).[1] Presumably any number of behavioral procedures could be used with selective mutism. Thus, many of the procedures used with language problem children (e.g., Gray & Ryan, 1973; Ruder, 1978; Schiefelbusch, 1978a, 1978b), autistic children (e.g., Lovaas & Bucher, 1974; Lovaas, Koegel, Simmons, & Long, 1973; Lovaas & Simmons, 1969), or noncompliant children (Kazdin, 1980a), could be utilized. The vast majority of reports in the selective mutism literature employed reinforcement procedures or other common operant techniques. The more common procedures are presented in Table 7.1.

---

[1]Many behavioral procedures have application to diverse behavior problems, as is demonstrated in the proliferation of differential attention applications over the past 20 years (cf. Hersen & Barlow, 1976).

TABLE 7.1
Basic Principles of Operant Conditioning

| Principle | Procedure | Behavioral Effect |
|-----------|-----------|-------------------|
| Positive reinforcement | Presentation of an event after a target response | Increased frequency of responding |
| Negative reinforcement | Removal of an event after a target response | Increased frequency of responding |
| Punishment | Presentation of an event after a target response | Decreased frequency of responding |
| Time-out | Removal of an event after a target response | Decreased frequency of responding |
| Extinction | Discontinuation of a reinforcing event after a target response | Decreased frequency of previously reinforced response |
| Stimulus control and discrimination training | Reinforcement of a target response in the presence of one stimulus ($S^D$) but not in the presence of another ($S^\Delta$) | Increased frequency of responding in the presence of the $S^D$ and decreased frequency of the response in the presence of the $S^\Delta$ |

*Reinforcement.* An event is regarded as a reinforcer if it increases the probability of the behavior it follows. Reinforcement can be either positive or negative. A *positive reinforcer* is an event that, when presented to the child, increases the behavior it follows. When removed it is called a *negative reinforcer*.

The use of reinforcement in the selective mutism literature was demonstrated when the therapist or teacher presented social or tangible events to increase the speech of the child. This procedure implies that these events are attrative to the child, but the real test of their effectiveness is the functional relation between the presentation and an increase in behavior. Reinforcement is a powerful behavior therapy procedure that has been demonstrated to be applicable across diverse settings and behaviors (e.g., Bandura, 1969; Krumboltz & Krumboltz, 1972; O'Leary & Wilson, 1975; Ullmann & Krasner, 1975).

*Punishment.* Whereas negative reinforcement involves the *removal* of a negative event contingent upon the presence of desirable behavior to be increased, punishment involves the presence of a negative event (aversive stimulus) contingent upon some undesirable behavior.[2] As is true of the reinforcement concept, the punishment principle specifies not only a procedure but

---

[2]Some authors also include response cost, or the reduction of a specific amount of reinforcement already present, as a punishment procedure (e.g., Goldfried & Davidson, 1976).

also the effect of that procedure on the target behavior. Generally, the two variations of punishment correspond to the variations of reinforcement. Behavior can be reduced in frequency by two procedures: the presentation of an aversive stimulus, or the removal of the client from a situation where he or she would typically be reinforced (i.e., time-out).

Several authors have employed either aversive procedures (e.g., Piersel & Kratochwill, in press) or time-out (e.g., Brison, 1966; Wulbert et al., 1973) in the treatment of selective mutism. For example, Wulbert et al. (1973) employed a time-out procedure in both experimental and control periods. If the child did not respond to a request for verbalization, he had to sit in the time-out room for 1 minute. Punishment is also a rapid and powerful procedure for changing behavior, but for practical and ethical reasons, it is frequently considered a method of last resort by some writers (Richards & Siegel, 1978). Indeed, it is possible that the use of punishment and other aversive procedures may account for much of the ethical concerns raised over behavior therapy in general (cf. Bandura, 1969; Krasner, 1971; Stolz et al., 1975). Some authors have suggested that aversive procedures are not the treatment of choice for children suffering from anxiety states and avoidance behavior, because they could produce or increase anxiety and avoidance (cf. Gelfand, 1979; Krumboltz & Krumboltz, 1972; Richards & Siegel, 1978). When aversive procedures are used, they can be combined with other treatment procedures such as reinforcement.

*Extinction.* In the extinction procedure, delivery of reinforcement occurs after some target response is discontinued. Whereas punishment involves an aversive event following a response or taking away a positive event (i.e., time-out), extinction requires that no consequence follow a target response. Thus, an event is not delivered or taken away (i.e., an event that was administered previously for the response is no longer provided). For example, Piersel and Kratochwill (in press) used extinction by having the teacher in the study ignore nonverbal communication. However, in their study, extinction was facilitated by simultaneously reinforcing the occurrence of an incompatible response (i.e., speech).

*Stimulus Control.* In an operant analysis, a response may be followed by a reinforcing or punishing consequence in the presence of one stimulus (labeled as $S^D$ or $S^+$) but not in the presence of another (labeled as $S^\Delta$ or $S^-$). Thus, a response reinforced in one situation but not in another situation comes under the control of the different situations. A situation previously associated with reinforcement of the target response will increase the probability that the response is performed when compared to the situation previously associated with no reinforcement. When a child has responded differentially to different stimuli, he or she has made a discrimination, and behavior is considered to be under stimulus control. For example, if a child's speech is reinforced in one situation (e.g.,

Classroom A) but not in another (e.g., Class room B), speech may come under control of the different classrooms. The classrooms (or their components, such as teachers) exert control over the verbal behavior because different reinforcement contingencies were associated with each stimulus situation.

*Other Operant Procedures.*    A variety of different concepts and variables have been employed in the operant literature, and many of them have been used in the treatment of mutism and other anxiety and avoidance behaviors (Richards & Siegel, 1978). *Shaping,* which refers to the gradual training of a complex response by reinforcing closer and closer approximations of it, was used by several writers (e.g., Bednar, 1974; Munford et al., 1976; Rosenbaum & Kellman, 1973; Sluckin & Jehu, 1969; Williamson et al., 1977a). In this strategy, the child is taught to elicit speech (words, phrases, sentences, and so on) by successive approximation. Such procedures as *fading* may also be employed. In teaching the mute child to speak, it is often useful at the beginning of the therapeutic program to utter a word loudly while encouraging the child to imitate. Over trials, the verbal prompt would then be faded, or gradually removed, as more normal speaking patterns are established. The steps used by Wulbert et al. (1973) in fading one experimenter into stimulus control of the mute child's verbal and motor behavior are presented in Table 7.2. During the experimental periods, the mother and child sat at a table in the clinic playroom. As the child responded appropriately to the task items administered by her mother, Experimenter 1 advanced through the successive steps of closeness described in Table 7.2.

*Modeling.*    Modeling is a behavior therapy procedure that refers to clients learning a desired response by observing the performance of the response by another person without performing it themselves. Modeling is sometimes called observational learning, vicarious learning, or imitation. Relative to many of the aforementioned operant techniques, modeling is a recent therapeutic technique, but it has been used in treatment of a variety of behaviors such as phobias and obsessions (see Bandura, 1971; Gelfand, 1979; Kirkland & Thalen, 1978; Rachman, 1972, 1976; Rosenthal, 1976; Rosenthal & Bandura, 1978; Zimmerman & Rosenthal, 1974). In the modeling strategy, the individual may observe a live or filmed performance of the model. A client may observe a significant individual or the self, as is characteristic of the self-modeling strategy.

Although many basic issues regarding its use as a therapeutic technique need to be resolved, basic laboratory research has suggested that such factors as similarity, status of the model, number of models, characteristics of the observer, and consequences following emulated behavior contribute to modeling effects (cf. Bandura, 1971; Kazdin, 1978a). Both a cognitive-mediational (Bandura, 1969, 1977b) and an operant paradigm (Gewirtz, 1971) have offered competing

TABLE 7.2
Graded Steps of Closeness Used in Fading Experimenter I
into Stimulus Control[a]

---

0. Neither visible nor audible.
   A. Neither visible nor audible.
   B. Not visible but audible over radio (saying "ask Emma question #1 or give Emma direction #17").
   C. Not visible but audible both over radio and from hall.
1. Visible at door.
   A. Visible and audible standing in hall, turned 180° away from Emma.
   B. Visible and audible standing in doorway, turned 180°.
   C. Visible and audible standing inside room with door closed, turned 180°.
   D. Visible and audible inside room, door closed, turned 135°.
   E. Visible and audible inside room, door closed, turned 90°.
   F. Visible and audible inside room, door closed, turned 45°.
   G. Visible and audible, facing with dark glasses on.
   H. Inside room with door closed, facing, radio off.
2. Inside room halfway to chair.
3. Inside room standing at chair.
4. Inside room sitting in chair.
5. Reading questions in unison with person already in stimulus control.
   A. Inside room reading task items in unison with mother and/or handing cards together.
   B. Inside room reading the critical element of the task item alone ınd/or handing cards together except mother drops hand before Emma takes.
   C. Inside room reading the crucial element of task alone, handing cards alone.
6. Reading questions alone while person in stimulus control remains seated at table.
   A. Inside room reading all the directions alone, holding and handing cards.
   B. Inside room, mother silent, but watching.
   C. Inside room, mother reading at table.
7. Reading questions alone while person in stimulus control moves away from the table.
   A. Inside room, mother reading with chair away from table.
   B. Inside room, mother reading with chair beside door.
   C. Inside room, mother in doorway.
   D. Inside room, mother in hallway.
8. Inside room, mother absent.

---

[a] Source: Wulbert, Nyman, Snow, and Owen (1973).

interpretations of modeling. Modeling has been used relatively infrequently in the treatment of selective mutism. Williamson et al. (1977a) used shaping with modeling as part of their therapeutic strategy. The child was instructed to imitate everything the therapist did with his mouth (e.g., blowing, "ah," "cat," and so forth). Nevertheless, modeling could be used more often in the treatment of selective mutism. Gelfand (1979) noted that with shy and withdrawn children, "effective modeling demonstrations have presented peer models as initially highly similar to the unskilled observers, but as increasingly assertive and successful [p. 38]." Gelfand (1979) also noted that shy children are best treated with modeling techniques in groups with normally assertive peers, rather than in groups that contain socially isolated children.

*Systematic Desensitization.*    Systematic desensitization is closely affiliated with the neobehavioristic mediational S–R model of behavior therapy (Kazdin & Wilson, 1978). Systematic desensitization typically involves three components (Kazdin & Wilcoxin, 1976). The client is first taught to relax, usually through some form of progressive relaxation training. Next, a hierarchy of stimuli are developed that represent the problem behaviors, such as a phobia, anxiety, or other problem. Stimuli composing these problems are typically ordered from least to most anxiety producing. Finally, while in a state of relaxation, the client is usually asked to imagine (or is shown) scenes in the hierarchy, beginning with the least provoking stimulus and gradually progressing through the hierarchy to the most provoking one. Typically, the client is not allowed to progress to a new hierarchy item until feeling comfortable with the prior item. In pairing relaxation with the hierarchy, the therapist assumes that anxiety will be inhibited through the principle of reciprocal inhibition.

Desensitization has been very effective in treating a wide range of problem behaviors such as fears, phobias, (e.g., illness, injury, death), obsessions and compulsions, depressions, and stuttering (cf. Bandura, 1969; Kazdin & Wilcoxin, 1976; Paul, 1969; Rachman, 1967).

Systematic desensitization has been applied, though infrequently, to the treatment of selective mutism (e.g., Scott, 1977). It appears that it could be applied to the problem with some advantage, particularly where severe anxiety accompanies the mutism. The therapist employing this procedure should consider the literature reviewing issues in its application (e.g., Jacobs & Wolpin, 1971; Kazdin & Wilcoxin, 1976).

*Mechanical Treatment Devices.*    Various technological developments have made it possible to employ a variety of instruments in psychotherapeutic work. In behavior therapy, a variety of mechanical instruments have found their way into treatment (see Rugh & Schwitzgebel, 1977; Schwitzgebel, 1976; for overviews). Schwitzgebel (1976) provided a classification of behavior modification devices that have been and can be used in behavior therapy. His eight classes of devices are briefly presented [p. 6]: The first class of devices are in a category called *frameworks.* Included here are static structures with passive control over space, light, sound, and/or temperature variables. Such devices (e.g., model lab) may be movable or changeable. *Hand tools* refer to devices with inert or rigidly related parts powered or operated by an individual. Scales used in a weight program represent an example of this category. A *reactive apparatus* refers to an assembly of movable parts powered by an individual with fixed mechanical output, typically with informational value (e.g., golf wrist counter). *Mechanical energy devices* refer to spring-driven apparatus that may or may not include an escapement mechanism used to release tension in equal units (e.g., timers). *Electromechanical or chemical devices* operate with a fixed or analogue output. They are typically powered by a battery or line current (e.g., electronic ear metronome for use in stuttering treatment). *Interdependent man–machine systems* refer to an array of interrelated human and electronic components with some human control of the apparatus output (e.g., shock device for writer's cramp). *Informational devices* are mechanical and electronic displays producing signals for information rather than work purposes (e.g., enuretic devices). Finally, *interactive information systems* refer to assemblages in which an apparatus (e.g., electrical) and an individual both act as subsystems with feedback control loops (e.g., teaching machines).

These various devices have been used in many areas of behavior therapy treatment and research. Any of the devices could be used in a treatment program for selective mutism, although very few studies have reported the use of such instruments. Nevertheless, some selective mutism researchers did use various devices to good advantage. For example, Nolan and Pence (1970) used a radio as a fading procedure to increase their client's voice loudness. Norman and Broman (1970) used visual feedback from a volume-level meter to induce sounds and raise speech volume. Blake and Moss (1967) employed a booth especially designed for autistic and mute children. Thus, some researchers employed various instrumentation devices or procedures in their overall treatment program to some benefit.

Although the device has not been used in any of the research reviewed in this text, Farrall Instruments has developed a puppet ("Gabby") that can be used with children who have trouble relating to adults and peers (see Fig. 7.1). The company notes that Gabby can be used in reduction of child–adult anxiety, elimination of speech defects, and for increasing verbalization.

*Package Programs.*    The conceptual framework for behavior therapy procedures can appear deceptively simple at first glance. Nevertheless, successful, effective implementation of these procedures requires careful training and skill. The reader unfamiliar with these procedures and behavior therapy in general is referred to several primary sources for detailed coverage (e.g., Goldfried & Davidson, 1976; Kazdin, 1980a; Mikulas, 1978; O'Leary & Wilson, 1975; Sulzer-Azaroff & Mayer, 1977).

Sometimes several independent therapeutic techniques are combined in the treatment of behavior disorders. Such a package denotes that several components of the treatment may be distinguishable on both conceptual and operational grounds (Kazdin & Wilson, 1978). For example, many researchers in the selective mutism area employed several specific therapeutic techniques in their therapy programs, such as prompting, modeling, instructions, feedback, reinforcement, and so forth. Usually, in the use of treatment packages, the primary

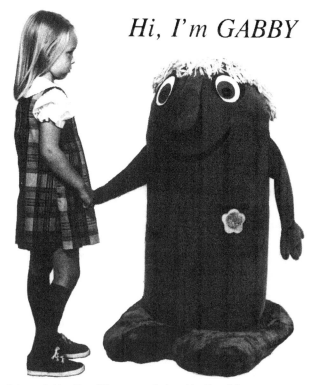

*Hi, I'm GABBY*

FIG. 7.1.   "Gabby," a talking puppet designed by Farrall Instruments, comes in three models. Gabby, Model F1, wireless-type talking puppet, is 38 inches high, weighs 95 pounds, is on a rocking base, and receives a communication from the loop system of any Farrall "Bug-in-the Ear" drivers. It is solid-state and is powered by 10 "D"-size batteries. Gabby, Model F1D is identical to the F1 but has a built-in edible dispenser that puts food into the puppet's pocket when a button on a remote-control unit is pushed. Gabby, Model F2, is identical to F1 but operates from an amplifier rather than the Bug-in-the-Ear system. Available from Farrall Instrument Company, P.O. Box 1037, Grand Island, Nebraska 68801. Reproduced by permission.

concern is with effecting rapid change in the client (Azrin, 1977). Although the package may contain many components, many may be unnecessary or even ineffective. Hopefully, the components will not neutralize each other's effects, although this may be a possibility. Thus, many of the aforementioned therapeutic techniques may be packaged where the primary concern is ameliorating the mutism.

Of course, use of a treatment package raises methodological concerns vis à vis identification of the active components responsible for the success of the program. However, applied psychologists are interested in outcome, or cure. In this context, the dimensions are clinical significance, speed, cost, generality, and degree of benefit (cf. Azrin, 1977). These are the activities for which practitioners are paid. In the context of treatment, Azrin (1977) noted:

> Only rarely have single-variable procedures been effective, most notably in decreasing by social extinction temper tantrums or other pure attention-getting behaviors. The criticism is frequently made of such "package" programs that one cannot identify which variable(s) is/are effective. My strategy has been to use such programs unapologetically and to include as many component procedures as seem necessary to obtain, ideally, a total treatment success. Once a treatment program is found to be extraordinarily successful, analytic studies of the program will be useful. But little seems to be gained by limiting oneself to partial benefits initially in order to achieve conceptual purity [p. 144].

In case therapists are interested in the evaluation of treatment packages, an evaluation scheme has recently been elucidated (cf. Kazdin, 1979; Kazdin & Wilson, 1978).

Recently, some package programs have been developed for the treatment of social withdrawal that can be useful in treating selective mutism. Such programs can be especially useful when the therapist finds that the client has many deficit behaviors in addition to the mutism. Hops, Walker and Greenwood, (1977) have described a program for remediating social withdrawal in the school setting. The program was developed at the Center at Oregon for Research in the Behavioral Education of the Handicapped (CORBEH). The center has specialized in the development of field-tested, packaged intervention programs for various types of excessive or deficient behavior problems frequently encountered in school settings (see Hops, et al., 1977).

The Program for Establishing Effective Relationship Skills (PEERS) contains a set of procedures for identifying and increasing the withdrawn student's positive social interactions with peers in playground and classroom settings. The program is implemented and supervised by a teacher-consultant and is managed in part by a classroom teacher and playground supervisor. Moreover, the total package contains procedures for brief training of teacher-consultants in using the interventions, thereby fulfilling a triadic intervention model (cf. Tharp & Wetzel, 1969).

More specifically, the PEERS program has been designed to use natural consequences for the peer environment to help the withdrawn child. The child is provided with the social skills necessary for admittance to the peer group via a social skills tutoring component. Backup reinforcement procedures are used to help assure that the peer group will accept the child. Moreover, a class and recess intervention program helps provide the child with opportunities to practice interacting both in free play and academic settings. Both self-report, verbal correspondence procedures, and fading components help to facilitate generalization and maintenance of therapeutic effects. Generally, the program appears to be quite successful for treating withdrawn children (see Hops et al., 1977, for an overview) and would likely be very useful in the treatment of selective mutism.

## PROCEDURES DESIGNED TO FACILITATE MAINTENANCE AND GENERALIZATION

As was suggested in Chapter 6, once an effective therapeutic procedure has been chosen, the therapist must still face the problem of durability and generalization of behavior change. A conventional notion of generalization is that it is a passive phenomenon. That is, it was not perceived as something to be programmed, but rather was the natural result of a behavior therapy program. However, the failure of responses to be maintained after a contingency is withdrawn (or to transfer across other settings) is to be expected on the basis of principles of operant conditioning (cf. Kazdin, 1978a). Because an assumption of the operant approach is that behavior is a function of its consequences, removal of these contingencies would adjust behavior to the removal. Although behavior changes made through operant techniques are not always lost when contingencies are removed, generalized and durable changes are typically exceptions.

Various research reports in the selective mutism literature assessed generalization but did not always program for it (e.g., Griffith et al., 1975). However, current knowledge in the field of behavior therapy indicates that not only should generalization be assessed; in addition, it should be actively programmed (Stokes & Baer, 1977; Wahler, Berland, & Coe, 1979). In recent years a number of authors have provided recommendations for facilitating maintenance and transfer
. of treatment results.

### Recommendations for Facilitating Maintenance and Transfer.

In Chapter 6 it was noted that generalization was an important feature of a behavior therapy treatment program. Although it has been uncommon to find researchers considering this aspect of treatment over the past few years, an embryonic technology for facilitating generalization has developed that is quite valuable in treating selective mutism. Authors have provided procedures that promote generalization in token reinforcement programs (e.g., Kazdin & Bootzin, 1972; O'Leary & Drabman, 1971; Wildman & Wildman, 1975), for psychotic patients (e.g., Liberman, McCann, & Wallace, 1976), and in general behavior therapy programs (e.g., Stokes & Baer, 1977; Sulzer-Azaroff & Mayer, 1977). Table 7.3 provides a general review of some procedures that have been identified as useful in facilitating generalization in behavior therapy.

Some specific procedures from the Stokes and Baer (1977) paper are reviewed because these techniques are quite useful to promote generalization of speech and

TABLE 7.3
Summary of Recommendations for Facilitating
Generalization from the Behavioral Literature[a]

| *Procedure* | *Source* |
| --- | --- |
| 1. Alter dimensions of reinforcement by: | |
| a. Fade or thin schedule | O'Leary and Drabman (1971) |
| | Kazdin and Bootzin (1972) |
| | Wildman and Wildman (1975) |
| | Sulzer-Azaroff and Mayer (1977) |
| | Kazdin (1978) |
| b. Decrease magnitude of reinforcement | Kazdin and Bootzin (1972) |
| | Wildman and Wildman (1975) |
| c. Increase delay of reinforcement | Kazdin and Bootzin (1972) |
| | Wildman and Wildman (1975) |
| | Kazdin (1978) |
| d. Substitute social reinforcement | Wildman and Wildman (1975) |
| | Kazdin (1978) |
| e. Substitute natural reinforcers | O'Leary and Drabman (1971) |
| | Liberman, McCann and Wallace (1976) |
| | Stokes and Baer (1977) |
| | Kazdin (1978) |
| 2. Choose small readily available reinforcers | Wildman and Wildman (1975) |
| 3. Choose behaviors that are: | |
| a. Selected by the subject | O'Leary and Drabman (1971) |
| b. Likely to be naturally reinforced later | Kazdin and Bootzin (1972) |
| | Wildman and Wildman (1975) |
| c. Functional | Liberman, McCann, and Wallace (1976) |
| d. Likely to bring subject into an environment where appropriate behavior will be reinforced | Wildman and Wildman (1975) |
| 4. Train in: | |
| a. Natural environment | Wildman and Wildman (1975) |
| | Kazdin (1978) |
| b. Environment similar to natural environment | Wildman and Wildman (1975) |
| c. Diverse environments | O'Leary and Drabman (1971) |
| | Liberman, McCann, and Wallace (1976) |
| | Sulzer-Azaroff and Mayer (1977) |
| | Stokes and Baer (1977) |
| | Kazdin (1978) |
| d. Presence of diverse stimuli | Kazdin and Bootzin (1972) |
| | Wildman and Wildman (1975) |

| Procedure | Source |
|---|---|
| | Sulzer-Azaroff and Mayer (1977) |
| | Kazdin (1978) |
| e. Environment with a number of individuals implementing the contingencies | Wildman and Wildman (1975) |
| 5. Decrease discrimination between reinforcement and nonreinforcement | O'Leary and Drabman (1971) Wildman and Wildman (1975) Stokes and Baer (1977) |
| 6. Use of common stimuli by: | |
| a. Emphasis on common elements | Sulzer-Azaroff and Mayer (1977) |
| b. Identification and use of discriminative stimuli | Sulzer-Azaroff and Mayer (1977) |
| c. Adding discriminative stimuli across situations | Sulzer-Azaroff and Mayer (1977) Stokes and Baer (1977) |
| 7. Involve the subject in: | |
| a. Selection of behavior | O'Leary and Drabman (1971) |
| b. Self-evaluation of behavior | O'Leary and Drabman (1971) Wildman and Wildman (1975) |
| c. Self-management | Kazdin and Bootzin (1972) Stokes and Baer (1977) |
| 8. Do not attempt generalization among incompatible behaviors by reinforcing only one of the behaviors | Wildman and Wildman (1975) |
| 9. Use level systems | Kazdin and Bootzin (1972) |
| 10. Look at school system as large token system | O'Leary and Drabman (1971) |
| 11. Teach child that achievement "pays off" | O'Leary and Drabman (1971) |
| 12. Give child the expectation that he can do well | O'Leary and Drabman (1971) |
| 13. Provide a good academic program | O'Leary and Drabman (1971) |
| 14. Teach controlling individuals in the environment how to maintain behavior | O'Leary and Drabman (1971) Kazdin and Bootzin (1972) Wildman and Wildman (1975) |
| 15. Train to generalize by reinforcing generalization behavior | Stokes and Baer (1977) |
| 16. Overlearn | Liberman, McCann, and Wallace (1976) |
| 17. Train sufficient exemplars | Stokes and Baer (1977) |
| 18. Train and "hope" | Stokes and Baer (1977) |

[a]Source: Miller (1978b).

language behavior (cf. Guess, Keogh, & Sailor, 1978). It should be remembered that these procedures can be helpful in facilitating both maintenance and transfer.

In their review of applied behavior research, Stokes and Baer (1977) noted that the procedures designed to assess or to program generalization can be loosely categorized according to seven general headings:

1. Train and hope.
2. Sequential modification.
3. Introduce to natural maintaining contingencies.
4. Train sufficient exemplars.
5. Train loosely.
6. Use indiscriminable contingencies.
7. Program common stimuli.

In their review, Stokes and Baer (1977) found that the most frequent treatments of generalization were also the least analytical (i.e., those described as "train and hope" and "sequential modification").[3] Train and hope involved those studies where the potential for generalization had been recognized and its presence or absence noted, but where no active attempt to establish generalization had been made. In sequential modification, given the absence of reliable generalization, procedures to effect changes were instituted directly in every nongeneralized condition. Unfortunately, these have not contributed to procedures that help to program generalization.

Stokes and Baer (1977) did review some categories that directly relate to a technology of generalization (see pp. 363–364). These include:

1. *Natural maintaining contingencies* wherein generalization may be programmed by suitable trapping manipulations, where responses are introduced to natural reinforcement communities that refine and maintain those skills without further treatment.

2. In *training sufficient exemplars,* generalization to untrained stimulus conditions and to untrained responses is programmed by the training of sufficient exemplars to those stimulus conditions or responses.

3. *Train loosely* is a programming technique in which training is considered with relatively little control over the stimuli and responses involved, and generalization is thereby enhanced.

---

[3]In the Stokes and Baer (1977) paper, some 270 applied behavior analysis studies relevant to generalization in that discipline were reviewed. Ninety percent of the literature reviewed was from five journals: *Behavior Research and Therapy, Behavior Therapy, Journal of Applied Behavior Analysis, Journal of Behavior Therapy and Experimental Psychiatry,* and *Journal of Experimental Child Psychology.* Seventy-seven percent of the literature reviewed was published since 1970.

4. In *indiscriminable contingencies,* reinforcement or punishment contingencies, or the setting events marking the presence or absence of those contingencies, are deliberately made less predictable, so that it becomes difficult to descriminate reinforcement occasions from nonreinforcement occasions.

5. *Common stimuli* are employed in generalization programming by incorporating into training settings those social and physical stimuli that are salient in generalization settings and that can be made to assume functional or obvious roles in the training setting.

6. *Mediated generalization* requires establishing a response as part of new learning that is likely to be utilized in other problems, also, and therefore to result in generalization.

7. *Train "to generalize"* involves reinforcing generalization itself as if it were an explicit behavior.

Stokes and Baer (1977) also suggest that these seven procedures contain a much smaller list of specific tactics. These include:

1. Look for a response that enters a natural community; in particular, teach subjects to cue their potential natural communities to reinforce their desirable behaviors.

2. Keep training more exemplars; in particular, diversify them.

3. Loosen experimental control over the stimuli and responses involved in training; in particular, train different examples concurrently, and vary instructions, $S^D_s$, social reinforcers, and backup reinforcers.

4. Make unclear the limits of training contingencies; in particular, conceal, when possible, the point at which those contingencies stop operating, possibly by delayed reinforcement.

5. Use stimuli that are likely to be found in generalization settings in training settings as well; in particular, use peers and tutors.

6. Reinforce accurate self-reports of desirable behavior; apply self-recording and self-reinforcement techniques wherever possible.

7. When generalizations occur, reinforce at least some of them at least sometimes, as if "to generalize" were an operant response class [p. 364].

These "what-to-do possibilities" can be used effectively in combination to promote maintenance and generalization of behavior change in the treatment of selective mutism. Of course, generalization will occur "naturally" (i.e., without active programming) in some instances, but more likely the therapist will need to rely on specific programming techniques. In future research on selective mutism, attempts should also be made to identify specific tactics that promote maintenance and transfer, so that these components can be added to the evolving technology of generalization (e.g., Sanok & Striefel, 1979).

## ETHICAL AND LEGAL ISSUES

This chapter has reviewed some behavior therapy techniques that can be useful in the treatment of selective mutism. Increasingly, legal and ethical issues have been considered in the application of therapeutic procedures, particularly due to some misuse of these treatment methods (Hare-Mustin, Marecek, Kaplan, & Liss-Levinson, 1979). Ethical principles have been advanced to promote the welfare of clients and to protect their rights. Various organizations have advanced standards for psychotherapeutic practice. For example, the *Ethical Standards of Psychologists* (American Psychological Association, 1977a) state: "Psychologists respect the dignity and worth of the individual and honor the preservation and protection of fundamental human rights [p. 1]." Moreover, the principles of medical ethics endorsed by the American Psychiatric Association (1973) ask psychiatrists to "render service to humanity with full respect for the dignity of man [*sic*]" and to "safeguard the public against physicians deficient in moral character or professional competence [p. 1059]." Other organizations such as the National Association of School Psychologists, the National Association of Social Workers (1967), and the Association for Advancement of Behavior Therapy also provide guidelines for professional practice.

In the use of specific therapeutic procedures such as those incorporated under the general rubric of behavior therapy, it is useful to distinguish between research and practice, although in many cases the same legal and/or ethical considerations may apply. A growing body of literature has addressed both research and treatment, ethical and/or legal considerations in the application of behavior modification techniques (e.g., Bersoff, 1978; Harris & Kapche, 1978; Kazdin, 1978a; Martin, 1975; Stolz, & Associates, 1978).

Martin (1975) presented a checklist that provides a useful scheme for instituting a behavior program:

1. Are the rules under which you operate written down in objective terms?
2. Are the individuals to be affected by a program given notice and an opportunity for a hearing?
3. Is the affected individual allowed the resources needed to challenge inclusion in the program if he wishes to do so?
4. Does the impact of inclusion in the program mean one group of individuals will be treated so differently from others that the distinction cannot be justified?
5. Does the participant in the program receive services in the same types of things which the institution generally provides, or does the program deprive the participants of something? If the latter, is it a constitutionally protected right or a privilege that is being withheld?
6. Is there an individual treatment program?
7. Are there periodic reviews of progress?
8. Is the least restrictive alternative explored first?

9. Are all the individuals in need of this program being offered services? If some are being excluded, can their separation be justified?

10. Is anyone's condition worsening?

11. Is anyone not receiving help because he has been assigned to a "control" group?

12. Is there a system in operation which allows those in charge to determine if something is wrong?

13. Have all funding agency guidelines been examined to determine if there are additional requirements [p. 10-11]?

One of the most extensive reviews of the ethical issues in behavior modification was presented by Stolz (1978). These authors reviewed the issues presented by the American Psychological Association Commission on Behavior Modification that are important in considering psychological interventions.[4] These include identification of the client, definition of the problem and selection of goals, selection of the intervention method, accountability, evaluation of the quality of the psychologist and the intervention, record keeping and confidentiality, protection of the client's rights, and assessment of the plan of research in therapeutic settings.

It was the commission's analysis of the advantages and disadvantages of having guidelines for the practice of behavior modification that led Stolz and Associates (1978) not to recommend the adoption of prescriptive and proscriptive guidelines.[5] Rather, the authors recommended: (1) that persons engaged in any type of psychological intervention subscribe to and follow the ethics, codes, and standards of their professions; and (2) that the APA consider adopting a brief checklist of issues that could be used in evaluating the ethics of any psychological intervention. They further suggested that the checklist be evaluated in practice and that the task of monitoring the evaluation be assigned to one of the APA's standing boards.

In this analysis, behavior modification procedures are treated as any other form of psychological intervention, with all procedures sharing similar ethical issues. In this regard, individuals would then follow the ethical codes and standards of their professions. For psychologists, these include the *APA's Ethical Standards of Psychologists: 1977 Revision* (1977a); the *Standards for Providers of Psychological Services* (APA, 1977b); a statement on psychology as a pro-

---

[4]Members of the APA Commission included Signey W. Bijou, Paul R. Friedman, James G. Holland, Leonard Krasner, Hugh Lavey, Stephanie B. Stolz, David Wexler, and G. Terence Wilson.

[5]This position contrasts to many reported in the literature (e.g., Agras, 1973; Harris & Kapche, 1978; Martin, 1975; Schwitzgebel, 1975). For example, Harris and Kapche (1978) provided guidelines for such problems as selection of the target child, data collection and record keeping, implementation of a behavior change program, and personnel qualifications.

fession (APA, 1968); *Ethical Principles in the Conduct of Research with Human Participants* (APA, 1973); and the *Standards for Educational and Psychological Tests* (APA, 1974). Of course, researchers and practitioners from other disciplines would follow their own standards (e.g., American Medical Association, American Psychiatric Association).

## SUMMARY AND CONCLUSIONS

In this chapter I suggested that attention to the various methodological and conceptual issues in the behavior therapy literature can be useful to both researchers and practitioners in the therapeutic field, especially those involved in treating selective mutism. Specific behavior therapy procedures were reviewed, with a special emphasis on procedures designed to facilitate maintenance and transfer of therapeutic gains. It was noted that some package programs designed for the treatment of social withdrawal may be especially useful in work on selective mutism. Ethical and legal issues remain as prominant concerns in therapeutic research and practice on childhood behavior disorders. Some guidelines for this endeavor were briefly presented.

# References

Achenbach, T. M. *Developmental psychopathology*. New York: Ronald, 1974.

Adams, H. B. "Mental illness" or interpersonal behavior? *American Psychologist*, 1964, *19*, 191-197.

Adams, H. E., Doster, J. A., & Calhoun, K. S. A psychologically based system of response classification. In A. R. Ciminero, K. S. Calhoun, & H. E. Adams (Eds.), *Handbook of behavioral assessment*. New York: Wiley-Interscience, 1977.

Adams, H. M., & Glasner, P. J. Emotional involvement in some form of mutism. *Journal of Speech and Hearing Disorders*, 1954, *19*, 59-69.

Adams, M. S. A case of elective mutism. *Journal of the National Medical Association*, 1970, *62*, 213-216.

Adkins, P. G. Tina talks. *Academic Therapy*, 1975, *11*, 91-96.

Adorno, T. W., Frenkel-Brunswik, E., Levinson, D. J., & Sanford, R. N. *The authoritarian personality*. New York: Harper & Row, 1950.

Agras, W. S. Toward the certification of behavior therapists. *Journal of Applied Behavior Analysis*, 1973, *6*, 167-171.

Albee, G. W. Conceptual models and manpower requirements in psychology. *American Psychologist*, 1968, *23*, 317-320.

Akler, H. A. Is personality situationally specific or interpsychically consistent? *Journal of Personality*, 1972, *40*, 1-16.

Allport, G. W. *Personality: A psychological interpretation*. New York: Holt, 1937.

American Psychiatric Association. *Diagnostic and statistical manual of mental disorders (DSM-I)*. Washington, D.C.: American Psychiatric Association, 1952.

American Psychiatric Association. *Diagnostic and statistical manual of mental disorders (DSM-II)*. Washington, D.C.: American Psychiatric Association, 1968.

American Psychiatric Association. *Diagnostic and statistical manual of mental disorders (DSM-III)*. Preliminary Edition, Washington, D.C., 1977.

American Psychological Association. *Ethical principles in the conduct of research with human participants*. Washington, D.C.: American Psychological Association, 1973.

American Psychological Association. *Standards for education and psychological tests.* Washington, D.C.: American Psychological Association, 1974.

American Psychological Association. *Ethical standards of psychologists: 1977 revision.* Washington, D.C.: American Psychological Association, 1977. (a)

American Psychological Association. *Standards for providers of psychological services* (Rev. ed.). Washington, D.C.: American Psychological Association, 1977. (b)

Amidon, E. The isolate in children's groups. *Journal of Teacher Education,* 1961, *12,* 412–416.

Amidon, E., & Hoffman, C. B. Can teachers help the socially rejected? *Elementary School Journal,* 1975, *66,* 149–154.

Amman, H. Schweigende Kinder. *Vierteljahresschrift für Heilpaedagogische und ihre Nachbargebiete* 1958, *27,* 209–216.

Appelman, K., Allen, K. E., & Turner, K. D. The conditioning of language in a nonverbal child conducted in a special education classroom. *Journal of Speech and Hearing Disorders,* 1975, *40,* 3–12.

Arajarvi, T. Elective mutism in children. *Annals of Clinical Research of the Finnish Medical Society* 1965, *11,* 46–52.

Arieti, S. (Ed.). *American handbook of psychiatry* (2 vols.). New York: Basic Books, 1959.

Arnold, G. E., & Luchsinger, R. *Lehrbuch der Stimm-und Sprach-Heipkunde.* Wien: Springer, 1949.

Aronson, A. E., Peterson, H. W., Jr., & Liten, E. M. Voice symptomatology in functional dysphonia and aphonia. *Journal of Speech and Hearing Disorders,* 1964, *29,* 367–380.

Aronson, A. E. Speech pathology and symptom therapy in the interdisciplinary treatment of psychogenic aphonia. *Journal of Speech and Hearing Disorders,* 1969, *34,* 321–341.

Asher, S., Oden, S., & Gottman, J. Children's friendships in school settings. In L. Katz (Ed.), *Current topics in early childhood education* (Vol. 1). Norwood, N.J.: Ablex Publishing Corp., 1977.

Austad, C. S., Sininger, R., & Stricklin, A. Successful treatment of a case of elective mutism. *The Behavior Therapist,* 1980, *3,* 18–19.

Axline, V. *Play therapy.* Boston: Houghton Mifflin, 1947.

Azrin, N. H. A strategy for applied research: Learning based but outcomes oriented. *American Psychologist,* 1977, *32,* 140–149.

Babcock, M. Speech therapy for certain vocal disorders. *Journal of Laryngology and Otolaryngology,* 1942, *62,* 101–112.

Baer, D. M. Perhaps it would be better not to know everything. *Journal of Applied Behavior Analysis,* 1977, *10,* 167–172.

Baer, D. M., Wolf, M. M., & Risley, T. R. Some current dimensions of applied behavior analysis. *Journal of Applied Behavior Analysis,* 1968, *1,* 91–97.

Bailey, J. S. *A handbook of research methods in applied behavior analysis.* Florida State University, 1977.

Bakwin, H., & Bakwin, R. M. *Behavior disorders in children.* Philadelphia: Saunders, 1972.

Baldwin, A. L. *Theories of child development.* New York: Wiley, 1967.

Bandura, A. A social learning interpretation of psychological dysfunctions. In P. Loudon & D. Rosenhan (Eds.), *Foundations of abnormal psychology.* New York: Holt, Rinehart & Winston, 1968.

Bandura, A. *Principles of behavior modification.* New York: Holt, Rinehart & Winston, 1969.

Bandura, A. Psychotherapy based upon modeling principles. In A. E. Bergin & S. L. Garfield (Eds.), *Handbook of psychotherapy and behavior change: An empirical analysis.* New York: Wiley, 1971.

Bandura, A. Self-reinforcement: Theoretical and methodological considerations. *Behaviorism,* 1976, *5,* 135–155.

Bandura, A. Self-efficacy: Toward a unifying theory of behavioral change. *Psychological Review,* 1977, *84,* 191-215. (a)

Bandura, A. *Social learning theory.* Englewood Cliffs, N.J.: Prentice-Hall, 1977. (b)

Bandura, A., & Walters, R. H. *Social learning and personality development.* New York: Holt, Rinehart & Winston, 1963.

Bangs, J., & Freidinger, A. A case of hysterical dysphonia in an adult. *Journal of Speech & Hearing Disorders,* 1950, *15,* 316-323.

Bannister, D., Salmon, P., & Leiberman, D. M. Diagnosis-treatment relationships in psychiatry: A statistical analysis. *British Journal of Psychiatry,* 1964, *110,* 726-732.

Barlow, D. H. Behavioral assessment in clinical settings: Developing issues. In J. D. Cone and R. P. Hawkins (Eds.) *Behavioral assessment: New directions in clinical psychology.* New York: Brunner/Mazel, 1977.

Barlow, D. H., & Hayes, S. C. Alternating treatments design: One strategy for comparing the effects of two treatments in a single subject. *Journal of Applied Behavior Analysis,* 1979, *12,* 199-210.

Barlow, R. A. A newer concept of functional aphonia. *Transamerican Laryngological Association,* 1930, *52,* 23-34.

Barton, R. T. The whispering voice syndrome of hysterical aphonia. *Annals of Otology, Rhinology, and Laryngology,* 1960, *69,* 156-164.

Bauermeister, J. M., & Jemail, J. A. Modification of elective mutism in the classroom setting: A case study. *Behavior Therapy,* 1975, *6,* 246-250.

Bednar, R. A. A behavioral approach to treating an elective mute in the school. *Journal of School Psychology,* 1974, *12,* 326-337.

Begelman, D. A. Misnaming, metaphors, the medical model, and some muddles. *Psychiatry,* 1971, *34,* 38-58.

Begelman, D. A. Ethical and legal issues of behavior modification. In M. Hersen, R. M. Eisler, & P. H. Miller (Eds.), *Progressive behavior modification* (Vol. 1). New York: Academic Press, 1976.

Bem, D. Constructing cross-situational consistencies in behavior: Some thoughts on Alker's critique of Mischel. *Journal of Personality,* 1972, *40,* 17-26.

Benassi, U., & Lanson, R. A survey of the teaching of behavior modification in colleges and universities. *American Psychologist,* 1972, *27,* 1063-1069.

Benjamin, L. S. Structural analysis of social behavior. *Psychological Review,* 1974, *81,* 392-425.

Bennett, P. S., & Maley, R. S. Modification of interactive behaviors in chronic mental patients. *Journal of Applied Behavior Analysis,* 1973, *6,* 609-620.

Bergan, J. R. *Behavioral consultant.* Columbus, Ohio: Charles E. Merrill, 1977.

Bergin, A. E., & Strupp, H. H. New directions in psychotherapy research. *Journal of Abnormal Psychology,* 1970, *76,* 13-26.

Bergin, A. E., & Suinn, R. M. Individual psychotherapy and behavior therapy. *Annual Review of Psychology,* 1975, *26,* 509-556.

Bersoff, D. N. Silk purses into sows' ears: The decline of psychological testing and a suggestion for its redemption. *American Psychologist,* 1973, *28,* 892-899.

Bersoff, D. N. Legal and ethical concerns in research. In L. Goldman (Ed.), *Research methods for counselors: Practical approaches in field settings.* New York: Wiley, 1978.

Bijou, S. W., & Grimm, J. A. Behavioral diagnosis and assessment in teaching young handicapped children. In T. Thompson & W. S. Dockens III (Eds.), *Applications of behavior modification.* New York: Academic Press, 1975.

Bijou, S. W., & Peterson, R. F. Functional analysis in the assessment of children. In P. McReynolds (Ed.), *Advances in psychological assessment* (Vol. 2). Palo Alto, Calif.: Science and Behavior Books, 1971.

Bijou, S. W., & Redd, W. H. Child behavior therapy. In S. Arieti (Ed.), *American handbook of psychiatry* (Vol. 5). New York: Basic Books, 1975.

Blake, P., & Moss, T. The development of socialization skills in an electively mute child. *Behavior Research & Therapy*, 1967, *5*, 349–356.

Blos, P., Jr. Silence: A clinical exploration. *Psychoanalytic Quarterly*, 1972, *41*, 348–363.

Bolgar, H. The case study method. In B. B. Wolman (Ed.), *Handbook of clinical psychology*. New York: McGraw-Hill, 1965.

Bonney, M. E. Assessment of effort to aid socially isolated elementary school pupils. *Journal of Educational Research*, 1971, *64*, 359–364.

Boone, D. Treatment of functional aphonia in a child and adult. *Journal of Speech & Hearing Disorders*, 1966, *31*, 69–74.

Brison, D. W. Case studies in school psychology. A non-talking child in kindergarten: An application of behavior therapy. *Journal of School Psychology*, 1966, *4*, 65–69.

Brodnitz, F. S. *Vocal rehabilitation*. Rochester, Minn.: American Academy of Ophthalmology, 1959.

Browne, E., Wilson, V., & Laybourne, P. Diagnosis and treatment of elective mutism in children. *Journal of the American Academy of Child Psychiatry*, 1963, *2*, 605–617.

Browning, R. M., & Stover, D. O. *Behavior modification in child treatment: An experimental and clinical appraoch*. Chicago: Aldine-Atherton, 1971.

Brunner, J. W., Goodnow, J. J., & Austin, G. A. *A study of thinking*. New York: Science Editions, 1965.

Calhoun, J., & Koenig, K. P. Classroom modification of elective mutism. *Behavior Therapy*, 1973, *4*, 700–702.

Callner, D. A. Behavioral approaches to drug abuse: A critical review of the research. *Psychological Bulletin*, 1975, *82*, 143–164.

Campbell, D. T., & Fiske, D. W. Convergent and discriminant validation by the multitract-multimethod matrix. *Psychological Bulletin*, 1959, *56*, 81–105.

Campbell, D. T., & Stanley, J. C. *Experimental and quasi-experimental designs for research*. Chicago: Rand McNally, 1966.

Carrier, J. K., & Peak, T. *Non-slip, non-speech language initiation program*. Lawrence, Kan.: H & H Enterprises, 1977.

Carson, R. C. *Interaction concepts of personality*. Chicago: Aldine, 1969.

Cartledge, G., & Milburn, J. F. The case for teaching social skills in the classrooms: A review. *Review of Educational Research*, 1978, *1*, 133–156.

Catania, A. C., & Brigham, T. A. *Handbook of applied behavior analysis: Social and instructional processes*. New York: Irvington Publishers, Inc., 1978.

Cautela, J. R., & Upper, D. *A behavioral coding system*. Paper presented at the meeting of the Association for Advancement of Behavior Therapy, Miami, December 1973.

Cerreto, M. C., & Tuma, J. M. Distribution of DSM-II diagnoses in a child psychiatric setting. *Journal of Abnormal Child Psychology*, 1977, *5*, 147–155.

Chapman, L. J., & Chapman, J. P. Sociatively based illusionary correlation as a source of psychodiagnostic folklore. In L. D. Goodstein & R. I. Lanyon (Eds.), *Readings in personality assessment*. New York: Wiley, 1971.

Chassan, J. B. *Research design in clinical psychology and psychiatry*. New York: Appleton-Century-Crofts, 1967.

Chetnik, M. The intensive treatment of an elective mute. *Journal of the American Academy of Child Psychiatry*, 1973, *12*, 482–498.

Ciminero, A. R. Behavioral assessment: An overview. In A. R. Ciminero, K. S. Calhoun, & H. E. Adams (Eds.), *Handbook of behavioral assessment*. New York: Wiley-Interscience, 1977.

Ciminero, A. R., Calhoun, K. W., & Adams, H. E. (Eds.) *Handbook of behavioral assessment*. New York: Wiley, 1977.

Ciminero, A. R., & Drabman, R. S. Current developments in the behavior assessment of children. In B. B. Lahey & A. E. Kazdin (Eds.), *Advances in child clinical psychology* (Vol. 1). New York: Plenum Press, 1977.

Clarizio, H. F., & McCoy, G. M. *Behavior disorders in children* (2nd ed.). New York: Crowell, 1976.

Clerf, L. F., & Braceland, F. J. Functional aphonia. *Annals of Otology, Rhinology and Laryngology*, 1942, *51*, 905-915.

Coates, T. J., & Thoresen, C. E. Using a generalizability theory in behavioral observations. *Behavior Therapy*, 1978, *9*, 605-613.

Coates, T. J., & Thoresen, C. E. Research on self-control. In D. C. Berliner (Ed.), *Review of research in education*. Itasca, Ill.: Peacock Publishers, 1979.

Cochrane, R., & Sobol, M. P. Myth and methodology in behavior therapy research. In M. P. Feldman & A. Broadhurst (Eds.), *Theoretical and empirical bases of the behaviour therapies*. London: Wiley, 1976.

Cole, L. E. *Understanding abnormal behavior*. Scranton, Pa.: Chandler, 1970.

Coleman, J. C., & Broen, W. E. *Abnormal psychology and modern life* (4th ed.). Glenview, Ill.: Scott, Foresman, 1972.

Colligan, R. W. Personal communication, 1978.

Colligan, R. W., Colligan, R. C., & Dilliard, M. K. Contingency management in the classroom treatment of long-term elective mutism: A case report. *Journal of School Psychology*, 1977, *15*, 9-17.

Cone, J. D. The relevance of reliability and validity for behavioral assessment. *Behavior Therapy*, 1977, *8*, 411-426.

Cone, J. D. The Behavioral Assessment Grid (BAG): A conceptual framework and a taxonomy. *Behavior Therapy*, 1978, *9*, 882-888.

Cone, J. D., & Hawkins, R. P. (Eds.). *Behavioral assessment: New directions in clinical psychology*. New York: Brunner/Mazel, 1977.

Conners, C. K. Symptom patterns in hyperkinetic, neurotic, and normal children. *Child Development*, 1970, *41*, 667-682.

Conrad, R. D., Delk, J. L., & Williams, C. Use of stimulus fading procedures in the treatment of situation specific mutism: A case study. *Journal of Behavior Therapy and Experimental Psychiatry*, 1974, *5*, 99-100.

Cook, T. D., & Campbell, D. T. The design and conduct of quasi-experiments and true experiments in field settings. In M. D. Dunnette & J. P. Campbell (Eds.), *Handbook of industrial and organizational research*. Chicago: Rand McNally, 1976.

Craighead, W. E., Kazdin, A. E., & Mahoney, M. J. (Eds.). *Behavior modification: Principles, issues, and applications*. Boston: Houghton Mifflin, 1976.

Creer, T. L., & Miklich, D. R. The application of a self-modeling procedure to modify inappropriate behavior: A preliminary report. *Behavior Research and Therapy*, 1970, *8*, 91-92.

Critchley, M. Spastic dysphonia ("inspiratory speech"). *Brain*, 1939, *62*, 96-103.

Cromwell, R. L., Blashfield, R. K., & Strauss, J. S. Criteria for classification systems. In N. Hobbs (Ed.) *Issues in the classification of children*. (Vol. I) San Francisco: Jossy-Bass, 1975.

Cronbach, L. J. *Essentials of psychological testing* (3rd ed.) New York: Harper & Row, 1970.

Cronbach, L. J., Glaser, G. C., Nada, H., & Rajaratman, N. *The dependability of behavioral measures*. New York: Wiley, 1972.

Davidson, W. S. II, & Seidman, E. Studies of behavior modification and juvenile delinquency: A review, methodological critique, and social perspective. *Psychological Bulletin*, 1974, *81*, 998-1011.

Derschowitz, A. M. Dangerousness as a criterion for confinement. *Bulletin of the American Academy of Psychiatry and the Law*, 1974, *2*, 172-179.

Deutsch, A. *The mentally ill in America*. New York: Columbia University Press, 1946.

Dickson, C. R. Role of assessment in behavior therapy. In P. McReynolds (Ed.), *Advances in psychological assessment* (Vol. 3). San Francisco: Jossey-Bass, 1975.

Dimond, R. E., Havens, R. A., & Jones, A. C. A conceptual framework for the practice of prescriptive electicism in psychotherapy. *American Psychologist,* 1978, *33,* 239-248.

Dmitriev, V., & Hawkins, J. Susie never used to say a word. *Teaching Exceptional Children,* Winter 1973, *6,* 68-76.

Doke, L. A. Assessment of children's behavioral deficits. In M. Hersen & A. S. Bellack (Eds.), *Behavioral assessment: A practical handbook.* New York: Pergamon Press, 1976.

Dollard, J., & Miller, N. E. *Personality and psychotherapy.* New York: McGrawHill, 1950.

Dornbusch, S. M., Hastorf, A. H., Richardson, S. A., Muzzy, R. E., & Vreeland, R. S. The perceiver and the perceived: Their relative influence on the categories of interpersonal cognition. *Journal of Personality and Social Psychology,* 1965, *1,* 434-440.

Dowrick, P. W., & Hood, M. Transfer of talking behaviors across settings using faked films. In E. L. Glynn & S. S. McNaughton (Eds.), *Proceedings of the New Zealand Conference for Research in Applied Behavior Analysis.* Aukland: University of Auckland Press, 1978.

Edgington, E. S. Statistical inference from N = 1 experiments *Journal of Psychology,* 1967, *65,* 195-199.

Ehrsam, E., & Hesse, E. Educational considerations on elective mutism, II. *Zeitschrift fuer Kinderpsychiatrie,* 1956, *23,* 7-11.

Eisenberg, L. Child psychiatry: The past quarter century. *American Journal of Orthopsychiatry,* 1969, *39,* 389-401.

Elles, G. The mute sad-eyed child. *International Journal of Psychoanalysis,* 1962, *43,* 40-49.

Ellis, M. Remarks on dysphonia. *Journal of Laryngology and Otology,* 1959, *73,* 99-103.

Elson, A., Pearson, C., Jones, C. D., & Schumacher, E. Follow-up study of childhood elective mutism. *Archives of General Psychiatry,* 1965, *13,* 182-187.

Endler, N. S., Boulter, L. R., & Osser, H. (Eds.). *Contemporary issues in developmental psychology* (2nd ed.). New York: Holt, Rinehart & Winston, 1976.

Engelmann, S., & Bruner, E. *Distar reading I.* Chicago, Ill: Science Research Associates, 1974.

Engelman, S., Osborn, J., & Engelman, T. *Distar language I.* Chicago, Ill.: Science Research Associates, 1972.

Erikson, E. H. *Childhood and society* (2nd ed.). New York: Norton, 1963.

Etemad, J. G., & Szurek, S. A. Mutism among psychotic children. In S. A. Szurek & I. N. Berlin (Eds.), *Clinical studies in childhood psychoses: 25 years in collaborative treatment and research, the Langley Porter Children's Service.* New York: Brunner/Mazel, 1973.

Eysenck, H. J. *Behavior therapy and the neuroses.* Oxford: Pergamon Press, 1960.

Eysenck, H. J. (Ed.). *Experiments in behavior therapy.* Oxford: Pergamon Press, 1964.

Farina, A., & Ring, K. The influence of perceived mental illness on interpersonal relations. *Journal of Abnormal Psychology,* 1965, *70,* 47-51.

Ferster, C. B., & Perrot, M. C. *Behavior principles.* New York: Appleton-Century-Crofts, 1968.

Fineman, K. *Developing sounds and word approximations in a deaf mute through systematic visual stimulation.* Unpublished paper, 1966.

Fiske, D. W. The limits for the conventional science of personality. *Journal of Personality,* 1974, *42,* 1-11.

Fliess, R. Silence and verbalization. *International Journal of Psychoanalysis,* 1949, *30,* 21-30.

Franks, C. M. (Ed.). *Behavior therapy: Appraisal and status.* New York: McGraw-Hill, 1969.

Franks, C. M., & Wilson, G. T. (Eds.). *Annual review of behavior therapy: Theory and practice* (Vol. IV). New York: Brunner/Mazel, 1977.

Freedman, A. M., & Kaplan, H. I. (Eds.). *Comprehensive textbook of psychiatry.* Baltimore: Williams & Wilkins, 1967.

Freud, E. D. Functions and dysfunctions of the ventricular folds. *Journal of Speech and Hearing Disorders,* 1962, *27,* 334-340.

Freud, S. [*New introductory lectures in psychoanalysis*] (W. J. H. Sprott, trans.). New York: Norton, 1933.

Friedman, R., & Karagan, N. Characteristics in management of elective mutism in children. *Psychology in Schools*, 1973, *10*, 249–252.

Froeschels, E., Dietrich, O., & Wilhelm, J. *Psychological experiments in speech*. Boston: Expression Co., 1932.

Froschels, E. *Stimm und sprache in der heilpaedagogik*. Halle; East Germany: Marshold, 1926.

Froschels, E. Method of therapy for paralytic conditions of the mechanism of phonation. *Journal of Speech and Hearing Disorders*, 1955, *20*, 365–370.

Furster, E. Zur systematik des kindlichen mutismus. *Zeitschrift fuer Kinderpsychiatrie* 1956, *23*, 175–180.

Games-Schwartz, B., Hadley, S. W., & Strupp, H. H. Individual psychotherapy and behavior. *Annual Review of Psychology*, 1978, *29*, 435–471.

Garfield, S. L., & Kurtz, R. M. Clinical psychologists in the 1970's. *American Psychologist*, 1976, *31*, 1–9.

Geiger-Martz, D. Zur psychotherapie bei elektivem mutismus. *Zeitschrift fuer Kinderpsychiatrie*, 1951, *17*, 169–174.

Gelfand, D. M. Behavioral treatment of avoidance, social withdrawal and negative emotional states. In B. B. Wolman, J. Egan, & A. O. Ross (Eds.), *Handbook of treatment of mental disorders in childhood and adolescence*. Englewood Cliffs, N.J.: Prentice-Hall, 1979.

Gelfand, D. M., & Hartmann, D. P. *Child behavior analysis and therapy*. New York: Pergamon Press, 1975.

Gewirtz, J. L. The roles of overt responding and extrinsic reinforcement in "self"—and vicarious reinforcement phenomena and in "observational learning" and imitation. In R. Glaser (Ed.), *The nature of reinforcement: A symposium of the Learning Research and Development Center, University of Pittsburgh*. New York: Academic Press, 1971.

Glass, G. V., Willson, V. L., & Gottman, J. M. *Design and analysis of time-series experiments*. Boulder: University of Colorado Press, 1975.

Goffman, E. *Asylums*. Garden City, N.Y.: Doubleday, 1961.

Goffman, E. The inmate world. In T. Million (Ed.), Theories of psychopathology and personality. Philadelphia: Saunders, 1973.

Goldfried, M. R. Behavioral assessment in perspective. In J. D. Cone & R. P. Hawkins (Eds.), *Behavioral assessment: New directions in clinical psychology*. New York: Brunner/Mazel, 1976.

Goldfried, M. R., & Davidson, G. C. *Clinical behavior therapy*. New York: Holt, Rinehart & Winston, 1976.

Goldfried, M. R., & Kent, R. N. Traditional versus behavioral personality assessment. *Psychological Bulletin*, 1972, *77*, 409–420.

Goldfried, M. R., & Pomeranz, D. M. Role of assessment in behavior modification. *Psychological Reports*, 1908, *23*, 75–87.

Goldfried, M. R., & Sprafkin, J. N. *Behavioral personality assessment*. Morristown, N.J.: General Learning Press, 1974.

Gottman, J. M., & Glass, G. V. Analysis of interrupted time-series experiments. In T. R. Kratochwill (Ed.), *Single subject research: Strategies for evaluating change*. New York: Academic Press, 1978.

Gottman, J. M., & Leiblum, S. R. *How to do psychotherapy and how to evaluate it*. New York: Holt, Rinehart & Winston, 1974.

Gough, H. G. *Manual for the California Psychological Inventory* (Rev. ed.). Palo Alto, Calif.: Consulting Psychologists Press, 1969.

Gray, B. F., England, G., & Mahoney, J. Treatment of benign vocal nodules by reciprocal inhibition. *Behavior Research & Therapy*, 1965, *3*, 187–193.

Gray, B. F., & Ryan, B. P. *A language program for the nonlanguage child.* Champaign, Ill.: Research Press, 1973.

Griffith, E. E., Schnelle, J. F., McNees, M. P., Bissinger, C., & Huff, T. M. Elective mutism in a first-grader: The remediation of a complex behavioral problem. *Journal of Abnormal Child Psychology,* 1975, *3,* 127–134.

Guerney, B. F., Jr., & Flumen, A. B. Teachers as psychotherapeutic agents for withdrawn children. *Journal of School Psychology,* 1970, *8,* 107–113.

Guess, D., Keogh, W., & Sailor, W. Generalization of speech and language behavior. In R. L. Schiefelbush (Ed.), *Bases of language intervention.* Baltimore: University Park Press, 1978.

Guess, D., Sailor, W., & Baer, D. M. *Functional speech and language training for the severely handicapped* (Parts I and II). Lawrence, Kans.: H & H Enterprises, 1977.

Gutzmann, H. *Vorlesungen ueber stoerungen der sprache und ihre heilung.* Berlin: Kornfeld, 1893.

Gutzmann, H. *Vorlesungen ueber spracheilkunde.* Berlin: Fisher, 1912.

Hall, C. S., & Lindzey, G. *Theories of personality.* New York: Wiley, 1970.

Hall, R. V., & Fox, R. G. Changing-criterion designs: An alternative applied behavior analysis procedure. In B. C. Etzel, J. M. LeBlanc, & D. M. Baer (Eds.), *New developments in behavioral research: Theory, Method, and application, In honor of Sidney W. Bijou.* Hillsdale, N.J.: Lawrence Erlbaum Associates, 1977.

Halpern, W. I., Hammond, J., & Cohen, R. A therapeutic approach to speech phobia: Elective mutism reexamined. *Journal of the American Academy of Child Psychiatry,* 1971, *10,* 94–107.

Hare-Mustin, R. T., Marecek, J., Kaplan, A. G., & Liss-Levinson, N. Rights of clients, responsibilities of therapists. *American Psychologist,* 1979, *34,* 3–16.

Harris, A., & Kapche, R. Behavior modification in schools: Ethical issues and suggested guidelines. *Journal of School Psychology,* 1978, *16,* 25–33.

Harris, S. L. Teaching language to nonverbal children—with emphasis on problems of generalization. *Psychological Bulletin,* 1975, *82,* 565–580.

Hartmann, D. P., & Hall, R. B. A discussion of the changing criterion design. *Journal of Applied Behavior Analysis,* 1976, *9,* 527–532.

Hathaway, S. R., & McKinley, J. C. *Manual for the Minnesota Multiphasic Personality Inventory.* Minneapolis: University of Minnesota Press, 1943.

Heaver, L. Spastic dysphonia II. *Logos,* 1959, *2,* 15–24.

Heinze, H. Freiwillig schweigende kinder. *Zeitschrift fuer Kinderforschung,* 1932, *40,* 235–256.

Hersen, M. Historical perspectives in behavior assessment. In M. Hersen & A. S. Bellack (Eds.), *Behavioral assessment: A practical handbook.* New York: Pergamon Press, 1976.

Hersen, M., & Barlow, D. H. *Single case experimental designs: Strategies for studying behavior change.* New York: Pergamon Press, 1976.

Hersen, M., & Bellack, A. S. *Behavioral assessment: A practical handbook.* Oxford: Pergamon Press, 1976.

Heuger, M. G., & Morgenstern, Mme. Un cas to mutisme chez un enfant myopathique ancien convulsif. Gnerion dn. mutisme par la psychoanalyse. *L'Encephale,* 1927, *22,* 478–481.

Hogan, R., DeSota, C. B., & Solano, C. Traits, tests, and personality research. *American Psychologist,* 1977, *32,* 255–264.

Holt, R. R. Yet another look at clinical and statistical prediction: Or, is clinical psychology worth while? *American Psychologist,* 1970, *25,* 337–349.

Holzberg, J. D. Reliability re-examined. In M. A. Richkers-Ovsiankina (Ed.) *Rorschach Psychology.* New York: Wiley, 1960.

Hops, H., Walker, H. M., & Greenwood, C. R. *Peers: A program for remediating social withdrawal in the school setting: Aspects of a research and development process* (Report No. 33). Eugene: University of Oregon Behavioral Education of the Handicapped Center on Human Development, 1590 Willamette Street, Eugene, Oregon 97401, 1977.

Howard, M. Art: A therapeutic tool. *Journal of the Oklahoma State Medical Association*, 1963, *56*, 420–424.

Isaacs, W., Thomas, J., & Goldiamond, I. Application of operant conditioning to reinstate verbal behavior in mute psychotics. *Journal of Speech and Hearing Disorders*, 1960, *25*, 8–12.

Jackson, C., & Jackson, C. L. Dysphonia plical ventricularis phonation with ventricular bands, *Archives of Otolaryngology*, 1935, *21*, 157–167.

Jackson, D. A., & Wallace, R. F. The modification and generalization of voice loudness in a fifteen-year-old retarded girl. *Journal of Applied Behavior Analysis*, 1974, *7*, 461–471.

Jacobs, A., & Wolpin, M. A. A second look at systematic desensitization. In A. Jacobs & L. B. Sachs (Eds.), *The psychology of private events: Perspectives on covert response systems*. New York: Academic Press, 1971.

Jensen, A. R. How much can we boost IQ and scholastic achievement? *Harvard Educational Review*, 1969, *39*, 1–123.

Johnson, S. M., & Bolstad, O. D. Methodological issues in naturalistic observation: Some problems and solutions for field research. In L. D. Harnerlynch, L. C. Handy, & E. J. Mash (Eds.), *Behavior change: Methodology, concepts, and practice*. Champaign, Ill.: Research Press, 1973.

Jones, R. R. Initial book review of single case experimental designs: Strategies for studying behavior change by Michel Hersen and David H. Barlow. *Journal of Applied Behavior Analysis*, 1978, *11*, 309–313.

Jones, R. R., Kanouse, D. E., Kelley, H. H., Nisbett, R. E., Valins, S., & Weiner, B. *Attribution: Perceiving the causes of behavior*. Morristown, N.J.: General Learning Press, 1971.

Jones, R. R., Reid, J. B., & Patterson, G. R. Naturalistic observation in clinical assessment. In P. McReynolds (Ed.), *Advances in psychological assessment* (Vol. 3). San Francisco: Jossey-Bass, 1975.

Kanfer, F. H., & Phillips, J. S. *Learning foundations of behavior therapy*. New York: Wiley, 1970.

Kanfer, F. H., & Saslow, G. Behavioral analysis: An alternative to diagnostic classification. *Archives of General Psychiatry*, 1965, *12*, 529–538.

Kanfer, F. H., & Saslow, G. Behavioral diagnosis. In C. M. Franks (Ed.), *Behavior therapy: Appraisal and status*. New York: McGraw-Hill, 1969.

Kanner, L. *Child psychiatry*. Springfield, Ill.: Charles C Thomas, 1975.

Kaplan, S. L., & Escoll, P. Treatment of two silent adolescent girls. *Journal of the American Academy of Child Psychiatry*, 1973, *12*, 59–71.

Kass, W., Gillman, A. E., Mattis, S., Klugman, E., & Jacobson, B. J. Treatment of selective mutism in a blind child: School and clinic collaboration. *American Journal of Orthopsychiatry*, 1967, *37*, 215–216.

Kazdin, A. E. Methodological and assessment considerations in evaluating reinforcement programs in applied settings. *Journal of Applied Behavior Analysis*, 1973, *6*, 517–531. (a)

Kazdin, A. E. Role of instructions and reinforcement in behavior changes in token reinforcement programs. *Journal of Educational Psychology*, 1973, *64*, 63–71. (b)

Kazdin, A. E. *Behavior modification in applied settings*. Homewood, Ill.: Dorsey Press, 1975.

Kazdin, A. E. Statistical analysis of single-case experimental designs. In M. Hersen & D. Barlow (Eds.), *Single case experimental designs: Strategies for studying behavior change*. New York: Pergamon Press, 1976.

Kazdin, A. E. Artifact, bias, and complexity of assessment: The ABC's of reliability. *Journal of Applied Behavior Analysis*, 1977, *10*, 141–150. (a)

Kazdin, A. E. Assessing the clinical or applied importance of behavior change through social validation. *Behavior Modification*, 1977. (b)

Kazdin, A. E. *History of behavior modification: Experimental foundations of contemporary research*. Baltimore: University Park Press, 1978. (a)

Kazdin, A. E. Methodology of applied behavior analysis. In T. Brigham & A. C. Catania (Eds.), *Handbook of applied behavior research: Social and instructional processes*. New York: Irvington Press/Halstead Press, 1978. (b)

Kazdin, A. E. Therapy outcome questions requiring control of credibility and treatment-generated expectancies. *Behavior Therapy*, 1979, *10*, 81-93.

Kazdin, A. E. *Behavior modification in applied settings (Rev. Ed.)*. Homewood, Ill.: The Dorsey Press, 1980. (a)

Kazdin, A. E. *Research design in clinical psychology*. New York: Harper & Row, 1980. (b)

Kazdin, A. E., & Bootzin, R. R. The token economy: An evaluative review. *Journal of Applied Behavior Analysis*, 1972, *5*, 343-372.

Kazdin, A. E., & Hartmann, D. P. The simultaneous-treatment design. *Behavior Therapy*, 1978, *9*, 912-922.

Kazdin, A. E., & Marholin, D. II Program evaluation in clinical and community settings. In D. Marholin II (Ed.), *Child behavior therapy*. New York: Gardner Press, 1978.

Kazdin, A. E., & Wilcoxin, L. A. Systematic desensitization and nonspecific treatment effects: A methodological evaluation. *Psychological Bulletin*, 1976, *83*, 729-758.

Kazdin, A. E., & Wilson, G. T. *Evaluation of behavior therapy: Issues, evidence, and research strategies*. Cambridge, Mass.: Ballinger, 1978.

Keeley, S. M., Shemberg, K. M., & Carbonell, J. Operant clinical intervention: Behavior management or beyond: Where are the data? *Behavior Therapy*, 1976, *7*, 292-305.

Keller, F. S., & Schoenfeld, W. N. *Principles of psychology*. New York: Appleton-Century-Crofts, 1950.

Kelly, G. A. *The psychology of personal constructs*. New York: Norton, 1955.

Kent, R. N., & Foster, S. L. Direct observation procedures: Methodological issues in naturalistic settings. In A. R. Ciminero, K. S. Calhoun, & H. E. Adams (Eds.), *Handbook of behavioral assessment*. New York: Wiley Interscience, 1977.

Kiml, J. Le classement des aphonics spastiques. *Folia Phoniatrica*, 1963, *15*, 269-277.

Kirkland, K. D., & Thalen, M. H. Uses of modeling in child treatment. In B. B. Lahey & A. R. Kazdin (Eds.), *Advances in child clinical psychology* (Vol. 1). New York: Plenum Press, 1978.

Kistler, K. Ein bemerksweter fall von freiwilligem schweigen im kindesalter. *Zeitschrift für Kinderforschung*, 1927, *33*, 2-14.

Klopfer, W. E., & Taulbee, E. S. Projective tests. *Annual Review of Psychology*, 1976, *27*, 543-567.

Koch, M. Elective mutism in children: A follow-up study. *Mental Health in Children*, 1976, *3*, 405-415.

Koch, M., & Goodland, L. Children who refuse to talk: A follow-up study. *Bulletin of the Bell Museum of Pathobiology*, 1973, *2*, 30-32.

Krasner, L. Behavior therapy. *Annual Review of Psychology*, 1971, *22*, 483-532.

Krasner, L., & Ullmann, L. P. *Behavior influence and personality: The social matrix of human action*. New York: Holt, Rinehart & Winston, 1973.

Kratochwill, T. R. *Single subject research: Strategies for evaluating change*. New York: Academic Press, 1978.

Kratochwill, T. R. Intensive research: A review of methodological issues in clinical, school, and counseling psychology. In D. C. Berliner (Ed.), *Review of research in education*. Itasca, Ill.: Peacock, 1979.

Kratochwill, T. R. Advances in behavioral assessment. In C. R. Reynolds & T. B. Gutkin (Eds.), *Handbook of school psychology*. New York: Wiley, 1981.

Kratochwill, T. R., & Bergan, J. R. Evaluating programs in applied settings through behavioral consultation. *Journal of School Psychology*, 1978, *16*, 375-386.

Kratochwill, T. R., & Brody, G. H. Single subject designs: A perspective on the controversy over employing statistical inferences and implications for research and training in behavior modification. *Behavior Modification,* 1978, *2,* 291-307.

Kratochwill, T. R., Brody, G. H., & Piersel, W. C. Elective mutism in children: A review of treatment and research. In B. Lahey and A. E. Kazdin (Eds.), *Advances in clinical child psychology.* New York: Plenum Press, 1979.

Kratochwill, T. R., & Levin, J. R. What time-series designs may have to offer educational research. *Contemporary Educational Psychology.* 1979, *3,* 273-329.

Kratochwill, T. R., & Wetzel, R. J. Observer agreement, credibility, and judgement: Some considerations in presenting observer agreement data. *Journal of Applied Behavior Analysis,* 1977, *10,* 133-139.

Krug, S. E. The role of personality assessment in the schools: A conversation with Dr. Raymond B. Cattell. *School Psychology Digest,* 1978, *7,* 26-35.

Krumboltz, J. D., & Krumboltz, H. B. *Changing children's behavior.* Englewood Cliffs, N.J.: Prentice-Hall, 1972.

Krumboltz, J. D., & Thoresen, C. E. (Eds.). *Counseling methods.* New York: Holt, Rinehart & Winston, 1976.

Kummer, R. Betrachtungen zum problem des freiwilligen schweigens. *Psychiatrie Neurologie und Medizinische Psychologie,* 1953, *5,* 79-83.

Kussmaul, A. *Die stoerungen der sprache.* Leipzig: Vogel, 1885.

Laing, R. D. *The politics of experience.* New York: Pantheon, 1967.

Landgarten, H. Art therapy as primary mode of treatment for an elective mute. *American Journal of Art Therapy,* 1975, *14,* 121-125.

Landgarten, H. Personal communication, 1978.

Lang, P. J. Fear reduction and fear behavior: Problems in treating a construct. In J. M. Schlien (Ed.), *Research in psychotherapy* (Vol. III). Washington, D.C.: American Psychological Association, 1968.

Lang, P. J. The application of psychophysiological methods to the study of psychotherapy and behavior modification. In A. E. Bergin & S. L. Garfield (Eds.), *Handbook of psychotherapy and behavior change.* New York: Wiley, 1971.

Lang, P. J. The psychophysiology of anxiety. In J. Akiskal (Ed.), *Psychiatric diagnosis: Exploration of biological criteria.* New York: Spectrum, 1977.

Lapoure, R., & Mouk, M. A. Fears and worries in a representative sample of children. *American Journal of Orthopsychiatry,* 1959, *29,* 803-819.

Lapoure, R., & Mouk, M. A. Behavior deviations in a representative sample of children. Variation by sex, age, race, social class and family size. *American Journal of Orthopsychiatry,* 1964, *34,* 436-446.

Laybourne, P. C., Jr. Elective mutism. In J. D. Noshpitz (Ed.), *Basic handbook of child psychiatry.* New York: Basic Books, 1979.

Lazarus, A. A. Has behavior therapy outlived its usefulness? *American Psychologist,* 1977, *32,* 550-554.

Lazarus, A. A., & Davidson, G. C. Clinical innovation in research and practice. In A. E. Bergin & S. L. Garfield (Eds.), *Handbook of psychotherapy and behavior change: An empirical analysis.* New York: Wiley, 1971.

Leventhal, T., & Sills, M. Self-image and school phobia. *American Journal of Orthopsychiatry,* 1964, *34,* 685-695.

Leitenberg, H. The use of single-case methodology in psychotherapy research. *Journal of Abnormal Psychology,* 1973, *82,* 87-101.

Lerea, L., & Ward, B. Speech avoidance among children with oral-communication defects. *Journal of Psychology,* 1965, *60,* 265-270.

Lesch, E. Ueber einen fall von freiwilligem schweigen. *Bericht ueber die 4. Versammlung der Deutsch Ges. Sprach-u. Stimmhk.* Berlin: Koblenz, 1934.

Levin, J. R., Marascuilo, L. A., & Hubert, L. J. Nonparametric randomization tests. In T. R. Kratochwill (Ed.), *Single subject research: Strategies for evaluating change.* New York: Academic Press, 1978.

Levy, M. P., & Fox, H. M. Psychological testing is alive and well. *Professional Psychology,* 1975, *6,* 420-424.

Liberman, R. P., McCann, M. J., & Wallace, C. J. Generalization of behavior therapy with psychotics. *British Journal of Psychiatry,* 1976, *129,* 490-496.

Liebmann, A. *Verlesungen ueber sprachstoerungen.* Berlin: Koblenz, 1898.

London, P., & Rosenhan, D. (Eds.). *Foundations of abnormal psychology.* New York: Holt, 1969.

Louttit, C. M., & Browne, C. E. The use of psychometric instruments in psychological clinics. *Journal of Consulting Psychology,* 1947, *11,* 49-54.

Lovaas, O. I., Berberich, J. P., Perloff, B. F., & Schaeffer, B. Acquisition of imitative speech by schizophrenic children. *Science,* 1966, *51,* 705-707.

Lovaas, O. I., & Bucher, B. D. (Eds.). *Perspectives in behavior modification with deviant children.* Englewood Cliffs, N.J.: Prentice-Hall, 1974.

Lovaas, O. I., Koegel, R., Simmons, J. Q., & Long, J. S. Some generalization and follow-up measures on autistic children in behavior therapy. *Journal of Applied Behavior Analysis,* 1973, *6,* 131-166.

Lovaas, O. I., & Simmons, J. Q. Manipulation of self-destruction in three retarded children. *Journal of Applied Behavior Analysis,* 1969, *2,* 143-157.

Lubin, B., Wallis, R. R., & Paine, C. Patterns of psychological test usage in the United States: 1935-1969. *Professional Psychology,* 1971, *2,* 70-74.

Macmahon, C. Treatment of functional aphonia. *Journal of Laryngology and Otology.* 1932, *47,* 243-246.

Mahoney, M. J. *Cognition and behavior modification.* Cambridge, Mass.: Ballinger, 1974.

Mahoney, M. J., & Arnkoff, D. Cognitive and self-control therapies. In S. L. Garfield & A. E. Bergan (Eds.), *Handbook of psychotherapy and behavior change* (2nd ed.). New York: Wiley, 1978.

Mahoney, M. J., & Thoresen, C. E. (Eds.). *Self-control: Power to the person.* Monterey, Calif.: Brooks/Cole, 1974.

Maloney, D. M., Harper, T. M., Braukmann, C. J., Fixsen, D. L., Phillips, E. L., & Wolf, M. M. Teaching conversation-related skills to pre-delinquent girls. *Journal of Applied Behavior Analysis,* 1976, *9,* 371.

Marholin, D. II (Ed.). *Child behavior therapy.* New York: Gardner Press, 1978.

Marholin, D. II, & Bijou, S. W. Behavioral assessment: Listen when the data speak. In D. Marholin II (Ed.), *Child behavior therapy.* New York: Gardner Press, 1978.

Marholin, D. II, Siegel, L. J., & Phillips, D. Treatment and transfer: A search for empirical procedures. In M. Hersen, R. M. Eisler, & P. M. Miller (Eds.), *Progress in behavior modification* (Vol. 3). New York: Academic Press, 1976.

Marks, I. M. *Fears and phobias.* New York: Academic Press, 1969.

Marshall, R. C., & Watts, M. T. Behavioral treatment of functional aphonia. *Journal of Behaviour Therapy and Experimental Psychiatry,* 1975, *6,* 75-78.

Martin, R. *Legal challenges to behavior modification.* Champaign, Ill.: Research Press, 1975.

Mash, E. J., & McElwee, J. Situational effects on observer accuracy: Behavioral predictability, prior experience, and complexity of coding categories. *Child Development,* 1974, *45,* 367-377.

Mayer-Gross, W., Slater, E., & Roth, M. *Clinical psychiatry* (3rd ed.). Baltimore: Williams & Wilkins, 1969.

McClelland, D. C., Atkinson, J. W., Clark, R. A., & Lowell, E. L. *The achievement motive.* New York: Appleton-Century-Crofts, 1953.

McCully, R. S. Current attitudes about projective techniques in APA-approved internship training centers. *Journal of Projective Techniques & Personality Assessment,* 1965, *27,* 271-280.

McLemore, C. W., & Benjamin, L. S. Whatever happened to interpersonal diagnosis?: A psychosocial alternative to DSM-III. *American Psychologist,* 1979, *34,* 17-34.

McReynolds, W. P. Diagnostic and statistical manual of mental disorders (3rd ed.) and the future of clinical psychology. *JSAS Catalog of Selected Documents in Psychology,* 1978, *8,* 69. (Ms. No. 1734)

McReynolds, W. P. DSM-III and the future of applied social science. *Professional Psychology,* 1979, *10,* 123-132.

Meichenbaum, D. H. *Cognitive behavior modification.* New York: Plenum Press, 1977. (Originally published, 1974).

Mikulas, W. L. *Behavior modification.* New York: Harper & Row, 1978.

Miller, J. F. Assessing children's language behavior. In R. L. Schiefelbush (Ed.), *Basis of language intervention.* Baltimore: University Park Press, 1978. (a)

Miller, A. J. *Facilitating generalization across settings through the use of adults as common discriminative stimuli.* Unpublished dissertation. The University of Arizona, 1978. (b)

Miller, L. C., Barrett, C. L., & Hampe, E. Phobias of childhood in a prescientific era. In A. Davids (Ed.), *Child personality and psychopathology: Current topics.* New York: Holt, Rinehart & Winston, 1974.

Millon, T. *Modern psychopathology.* Philadelphia: Saunders, 1969.

Millon, T., & Millon, R. *Abnormal behavior and personality.* Philadelphia: Saunders, 1974.

Mischel, W. *Personality and assessment.* New York: Wiley, 1968.

Mischel, W. Direct versus indirect personality assessment: Evidence and implications. *Journal of Consulting and Clinical Psychology,* 1972, *38,* 319-324.

Mischel, W. Facing the issues. *Journal of Abnormal Psychology,* 1973, *82,* 541-542. (a)

Mischel, W. On the empirical dilemmas of psychodynamic approaches: Issues and alternatives. *Journal of Abnormal Psychology,* 1973, *82,* 335-344. (b)

Mischel, W. Toward a cognitive social learning reconceptualization of personality. *Psychological Review,* 1973, *80,* 252-283. (c)

Mischel, W. Cognitive appraisals and transformations in self-control. In B. Weiner (Ed.), *Cognitive views of human motivation.* New York: Academic Press, 1974.

Mischel, W. *Introduction to personality* (2nd ed.). New York: Holt, Rinehart & Winston, 1976.

Mitscherlich, M. Zwei faelle von psychogenem mutismus. *Zeitschrift fuer Psychosomatische Medizin und Psychoanalyse,* 1952, *7,* 172-175.

Mora, G. Personal communication, 1978.

Mora, G., Devault, S., & Schopler, E. Dynamics and psychotherapy of identical twins with elective mutism. *Journal of Child Psychology and Psychiatry,* 1962, *3,* 41-52.

Morris, J. Cases of elective mutism. *American Journal of Mental Deficiency,* 1953, *57,* 661-668.

Moss, T., & Blake, P. R. A dynamic-behavioral approach to therapy with an electively mute child: A follow-up study. In K. L. Beauchamp, R. L. Bruce, & D. W. Matheson (Eds.), *Current topics in experimental psychology.* New York: Holt, Rinehart & Winston, 1970.

Munford, P. R. Personal communication, June 15, 1978.

Munford, P. R., Reardon, D., Liberman, R. P., & Allen, L. Behavioral treatment of hysterical coughing and mutism: A case study. *Journal of Consulting and Clinical Psychology,* 1976, *4,* 1008-1014.

Nadoleczng, M. *Die sprachstoerungen im kindesalter.* Leipzig: Vogel, 1926.

Nash, R. T., Thorpe, H. W., Andrews, M. M., & Davis, K. A management program for elective mutism. Psychology in the Schools, 1979, *16,* 246-253.

Nay, W. R. Analogue measures. In A. R. Ciminero, K. S. Calhoun, & H. E. Adams (Eds.), *Handbook of behavioral assessment.* New York: Wiley, 1977.

Nolan, J. D. Personal communication, June 23, 1978.

Nolan, J., & Pence, C. Operant conditioning principles in the treatment of a selectively mute child. *Journal of Consulting and Clinical Psychology,* 1970, *35,* 265-268.

Norman, A., & Broman, H. J. Volume feedback and generalization techniques in shaping speech of an electively mute boy: A case study. *Perceptual and Motor Skills,* 1970, *31,* 463-470.

O'Connor, R. D. Modification of social withdrawal through symbolic modeling. *Journal of Applied Behavior Analysis,* 1969, *2,* 15-22.

O'Connor, R. D. Relative efficacy of modeling, shaping, and the combined procedures for modification of social withdrawal. *Journal of Abnormal Psychology,* 1972, *79,* 327-334.

O'Leary, K. D. The assessment of psychopathology in children. In H. C. Quay & J. S. Werry (Eds.), *Psychopathological disorders of childhood.* New York: Wiley, 1972.

O'Leary, K. D., & Drabman, R. Token reinforcement programs in the classroom: A review. *Psychological Bulletin,* 1971, *75,* 379-398.

O'Leary, K. D., & Johnson, S. B. Psychological assessment. In H. C. Quay & J. S. Werry (Eds.), *Psychopathological disorders of childhood* (2nd ed.). New York: Wiley, 1979.

O'Leary, K. D., & Kent, R. Behavior modification for social action: Research tactics and problems. In L. A. Hamerlynck, L. C. Handy, & E. J. Mash (Eds.), *Behavior change: Methodology concepts and practice.* Champaign, Ill.: Research Press, 1973.

O'Leary, K. D., & Wilson, G. T. *Behavior therapy: Application and outcome.* Englewood Cliffs, N.J.: Prentice-Hall, 1975.

Pangalila-Ratulangie, E. A. Clinical treatment of a case of mutism. *Zeitschrift für Kinderpsychiatrie,* 1959, *26,* 33-41.

Panzetta, A. F. Towards a scientific psychiatric nosology. *Archives of General Psychiatry,* 1974, *30,* 154-161.

Parker, E. B., Olsen, T. F., & Throckmorton, M. C. Social case work with elementary school children who do not talk in school. *Social Work,* 1960, *5,* 64-70.

Patterson, G. R. An application of conditioning techniques to the control of a hyperactive child. In L. Ullman & K. Krasner (Eds.), *Case studies in behavior modification.* New York: Holt, Rinehart & Winston, 1965.

Paul, G. L. Behavior modification research: Design and tactics. In C. M. Franks (Ed.), *Behavior therapy: Appraisal and status.* New York: McGraw-Hill, 1969.

Paul, G. L., & Bernstein, D. A. *Anxiety and clinical problems: Systematic desensitization and related techniques.* Morristown, N.J.: General Learning Press, 1973.

Pervin, L. A. *Personality: Theory, assessment, and research.* New York: Wiley, 1975.

Peterson, D. R. *The clinical study of social behavior.* New York: Appleton-Century-Crofts, 1968.

Phillips, L., & Draguns, J. G. Classification of the behavior disorders. *Annual Review of Psychology,* 1971, *22,* 447-482.

Phillips, L., Draguns, J. G., & Bartlett, D. P. Classification of behavior disorders. In N. Hobbs (Ed.), *Issues in the classification of children* (Vol. 1) San Francisco: Jossy-Bass, 1975.

Piersel, W. C., & Kratochwill, T. R. A teacher implemented contingency management package to treat selective mutism. *Behavioral Assessment,* 1981.

Pustrom, E., & Speers, R. W. Elective mutism in children. *Journal of the American Academy of Child Psychiatry,* 1964, *3,* 287-297.

Quay, H. C. Patterns of aggression, withdrawal, and immaturity. In H. C. Quay & J. S. Werry (Eds.), *Psychopathological disorders of childhood.* New York: Wiley, 1972.

Quay, H. C. Classification. In H. C. Quay & J. S. Werry (Eds.), *Psychopathological disorders of childhood* (2nd ed.). New York: Wiley, 1979.

Rachman, S. Introduction to behaviour therapy. *Behaviour Research and Therapy,* 1963, *1,* 4-15.

Rachman, S. Systematic desensitization. *Psychological Bulletin,* 1967, *67,* 93-103.

Rachman, S. Clinical applications of observational learning, imitation and modeling. *Behavior Therapy,* 1972, *3,* 379-397.

Rachman, S. J. Observational learning and therapeutic modeling. In M. P. Feldman & A. Broadhurst (Eds.), *Theoretical and empirical bases of the behavior therapies*. London: Wiley, 1976.

Rakoff, V. M., Stancer, H. C., & Kedward, H. B. (Eds.) *Psychiatric diagnosis*. New York: Brunner/Mazel, 1977.

Rasbury, W. C. Behavioral treatment of selective mutism: A case report. *Behavioral Therapy and Experimental Psychiatry*, 1974, *5*, 103-104.

Redd, W. H. Effects of mixed reinforcement contingencies on adults' control of children's behavior. *Journal of Applied Behavior Analysis*, 1969, *2*, 249-254.

Reed, G. F. Elective mutism in children: A re-appraisal. *Journal of Child Psychology and Psychiatry*, 1963, *4*, 99-107.

Reid, J. B., Hawkins, N., Keutzer, C., McNeal, S. A., Phelps, R. E., Reid, K. M., & Meas, H. L. A marathon behavior modification of a selectively mute child. *Journal of Child Psychology and Psychiatry*, 1967, *8*, 27-30.

Rhodes, W. C., & Paul, J. L. *Emotionally disturbed and deviant children: New views & approaches*. Englewood Cliffs, N.J.: Prentice-Hall, 1978.

Richards, C. S., & Siegel, L. J. Behavioral treatment of anxiety states and avoidance behaviors in children. In D. Marholin II (Ed.), *Child behavior therapy*. New York: Gardner Press, 1978.

Rigby, M. A case of lack of speech due to negativism. *Psychological Clinic*, 1929, *18*, 156-161.

Risley, T. R. Behavior modification: An experimental-therapeutic endeavor. In L. A. Hammerlynck, P. O. Davidson, & L. E. Acker (Eds.), *Behavior modification and ideal mental health services*. Alberta: University of Calgary, 1970.

Robins, L. N. Follow-up studies. In H. C. Quay & J. S. Werry (Eds.), *Psychopathological disorders of childhood*. New York: Wiley, 1979.

Robinson, P. W., & Foster, D. F. *Experimental psychology: A small-n approach*. New York: Harper & Row, 1979.

Rosenbaum, E., & Kellman, M. Treatment of a selectively mute third-grade child. *Journal of School Psychology*, 1973, *11*, 26-29.

Rosenhan, D. On being sane in an insane place. *Science*, 1973, *179*, 250-258.

Rosenthal, R., & Jacobsen, L. *Pygmalion in the classroom: Teacher expectations and pupils' intellectual development*. New York: Holt, 1968.

Rosenthal, T. L. Modeling therapies. In M. Hersen, R. M. Eisler, & P. M. Miller (Eds.), *Progress in behavior modification* (Vol. 2). New York: Academic Press, 1976.

Rosenthal, T. L., & Bandura, A. Psychological modeling: Theory and practice. In S. L. Garfield & A. E. Bergin (Eds.), *Handbook of psychotherapy and behavior change*. New York: Wiley, 1978.

Ross, A. O. *Psychological disorders of children: A behavioral approach to theory, research and therapy*. New York: McGraw-Hill, 1974.

Ross, A. O., & Nelson, R. O. Behavior therapy. In H. C. Quay & J. S. Werry (Eds.), *Psychopathological disorders of childhood* (2nd ed.). New York: Wiley, 1979.

Rothe, C. Sprachscheue kinder. *Z. Ohrenheilk.*, 1928, *62*, 904-909.

Ruder, K. F. Planning and programming for language intervention. In R. L. Schiefelbush (Ed.), *Bases of language intervention*. Baltimore: University Park Press, 1978.

Rugh, J. D., & Schwitzgebel, R. L. Instrumentation for behavioral assessment. In A. R. Ciminero, K. S. Calhoun, & H. E. Adams (Eds.), *Handbook of behavioral assessment*. New York: Wiley, 1977.

Rutter, M., & Hersov, L. *Child psychiatry: Modern approaches*. Oxford, England: Blackwell Scientific Publications, 1977.

Ruzicka, B., & Sackin, H. D. Elective mutism: The impact of the patient's silent detachment upon the therapist. *Journal of the American Academy of Child Psychiatry*, 1974, *13*, 551-560.

Salfield, D. J. Observations on elective mutism in children. *Journal of Mental Science,* 1950, *96,* 1024-1032.

Salfield, D. J., Lond, B., & Dusseldorf, M. D. Observations on elective mutism in children. *Journal of Mental Science,* 1950, *96,* 1024-1032.

Salzinger, K. A behavioral analysis of diagnosis. In R. L. Spitzer & D. F. Klein (Eds.), *Critical issues in psychiatric diagnosis.* New York: Raven Press, 1978.

Sandifer, M. G., Pettus, C., & Quade, D. A study of psychiatric diagnosis. *Journal of Nervous and Mental Disease,* 1964, *139,* 350-356.

Sanok, R. L., & Ascione, F. R. Behavioral interventions for childhood elective mutism: An evaluative review. *Child Behavior Therapy,* 1979, *1,* 49-68.

Sanok, R. L., & Striefel, S. *Elective mutism: Generalization of verbal responding across people and settings.* Behavior Therapy, 1979, *10,* 357-371.

Sarason, S. B. The unfortunate fate of Alfred Binet and school psychology. *Teachers College Record,* 1976, *77,* 579-592.

Sarbin, T. R., & Mancuso, J. C. Failure of a moral enterprise: Attitudes of the public toward mental illness. *Journal of Consulting and Clinical Psychology,* 1970, *35,* 159-173.

Schacht, T., & Nathan, P. E. But is it good for the psychologists? Appraisal and status of DSM-III. *American Psychologist,* 1977, *32,* 1017-1025.

Scheff, T. *Being mentally ill.* Chicago: Aldine, 1966.

Scheff, T. J. The role of the mentally ill and the dynamics of mental disorder. In T. Millon (Ed.), *Theories of psychopathology and personality.* Philadelphia: Saunders, 1973.

Schepank, H. Ein fall von elektivem mutismus in kindesalter. *Praxis der Kinderpsychologie und Kinderpsychiatrie* 1960, *9,* 124-137.

Schiefelbusch, R. L. (Ed.). *Basis of language intervention.* Baltimore: University Park Press, 1978. (a)

Schiefelbusch, R. L. (Ed.). *Language intervention strategies.* Baltimore: University Park Press, 1978. (b)

Schmidt, H. O., & Fonda, C. P. The reliability of psychiatric diagnosis: A new look. *Journal of Abnormal and Social Psychology,* 1956, *52,* 262-267.

Schnelle, J. F. A brief report on invalidity of parent evaluations of behavior change. *Journal of Applied Behavior Analysis,* 1974, *7,* 341-343.

Schwitzgebel, R. K. A contractual model for the protection of the rights of institutionalized mental patients. *American Psychologist,* 1975, *30,* 815-820.

Schwitzgebel, R. K. Behavioral technology. In H. Leitenberg (Ed.), *Handbook of behavior modification and behavior therapy.* Englewood Cliffs, N.J.: Prentice-Hall, 1976.

Scott, E. A desensitization program for the treatment of mutism in a seven-year-old girl: A case report. *Journal of Child Psychology and Psychiatry,* 1977, *18,* 263-270.

Sears, R. R., Rau, L., & Alpert, R. *Identification and child rearing.* Stanford, Calif.: Stanford University Press, 1965.

Seeman, W. P. Psychiatric diagnosis: An investigation of interpersonal-reliability after didactic instruction. *Journal of Nervous and Mental Disease,* 1953, *118,* 541-544.

Semenoff, B., Park, C., & Smith, E. Behavior interventions with a six-year-old elective mute. In J. D. Krumboltz & C. E. Thoresen (Eds.), *Counseling methods.* New York: Holt, Rinehart & Winston, 1976.

Shapiro, M. B. The single case in fundamental clinical psychological research. *British Journal of Medical Psychology,* 1961, *34,* 255-262.

Shapiro, M. B. The single case in clinical psychological research. *Journal of General Psychology,* 1966, *74,* 3-23.

Shaw, W. H. Aversive control in treatment of elective mutism. *Journal of the American Academy of Child Psychiatry,* 1971, *10,* 572-581.

Shemberg, K., & Keeley, S. Psychodiagnostic training in the academic setting: Past and present. *Journal of Consulting & Clinical Psychology*, 1970, *34*, 205-211.

Sherman, H., & Farina, A. Social inadequacy of parents and children. *Journal of Abnormal Psychology*, 1974, *83*, 327-330.

Sherman, J. A. Reinstatement of verbal behavior in a psychotic by reinforcement methods. *Journal of Speech and Hearing Disorders*, 1963, *28*, 398-401.

Sherman, J. A. Use of reinforcement and imitation to reinstate verbal behavior in mute psychotics. *Journal of Abnormal Psychology*, 1969, *70*, 155-164.

Shirley, H. F. *Pediatric psychiatry*. Cambridge, Mass.: Harvard University Press, 1963.

Sidman, M. *Tactics of scientific research: Evaluating experimental data in psychology*. New York: Basic Books, 1960.

Silverman, G., & Powers, D. G. Elective mutism in children. *Medical College of Virginia Quarterly*, 1970, *6*, 182-186.

Silverman, L. H. Psychoanalytic theroy: "The reports of my death are greatly exaggerated." *American Psychologist*, 1976, *31*, 621-637.

Skinner, B. F. *Science and human behavior*. New York: Macmillan, 1953.

Sluckin, A., & Jehu, D. A behavioral approach in the treatment of elective mutism. *British Journal of Psychiatric Social Work*, 1969, *10*, 70-73.

Smayling, L. M. Analyses of six cases of voluntary mutism. *Journal of Speech and Hearing Disorders*, 1959, *24*, 55-58.

Snow, R. E. Representative and quasi-representative designs for research in teaching. *Review of Educational Research*, 1974, *44*, 265-291.

Spieler, J. Freiwillige schweiger und sprachscheue kinder. *Zeitschrift für Kinderforschung*, 1941, *49*, 39-43.

Spieler, J. *Schweigende und sprachscheue kinder*. Olten, Switzerland: Otto Walter, 1944.

Spitzer, R. L., & Endicott, J. E. Medical and mental disorder: Proposed definition and criteria. In R. L. Spitzer & D. Klein (Eds.), *Critical issues in psychiatric diagnosis*. New York: Raven Press, 1978.

Spitzer, R. L., & Klein, D. F. *Critical issues in psychiatric diagnosis*. New York: Raven Press, 1978.

Spitzer, R. L., Sheehy, M., & Endicott, J. DSM-III: Guiding principles. In V. M. Rakoff, H. C. Stancer, & H. B. Kedward (Eds.), *Psychiatric diagnosis*. New York: Brunner/Mazel, 1977.

Spitzer, R. L., & Williams, J. B. W. Classification of mental disorders and DSM-III. In H. I. Kaplan, A. M. Freedman, and B. J. Sadock (Eds.), *Comprehensive textbook of psychiatry/III* (Volume 1). Baltimore: Williams and Wilkins, 1980.

Spitzer, R. L., & Wilson, P. T. Nosology and the official psychiatric nomenclature. In A. M. Freedman, H. I. Kaplan, & B. J. Sadock (Eds.), *Comprehensive textbook of psychiatry*. Baltimore: Williams & Wilkins, 1975.

Stern, H. Vortrag ueber die verschiedenen formen der stummheit. *Wiener Medizinische Wochenschrift*, 1910, *60*, 924-933.

Stokes, T. F., & Baer, D. M. An implicit technology of generalization. *Journal of Applied Behavior Analysis*, 1977, *10*, 349-367.

Stoller, R. J., & Geertsma, R. H. The consistency of psychiatrists' clinical judgments. *Journal of Nervous and Mental Disease*, 1963, *137*, 58-66.

Stolz, S. B., & Associates. *Ethical issues in behavior modification*. San Francisco: Jossey-Bass, 1978.

Stolz, S. B., Wienckowski, L. A., & Brown, B. S. Behavior modification: A perspective on critical issues. *American Psychologist*, 1975, *30*, 1027-1048.

Strain, P. S., Cooke, T. P., & Apolloni, T. *Teaching exceptional children: Assessing and modifying social behavior*. New York: Academic Press, 1976.

Strait, R. A child who was speechless in school and social life. *Journal of Speech and Hearing Disorders*, 1958, *23*, 253–254.

Straughan, J. H. The application of operant conditioning to the treatment of elective mutism. In H. Sloane & B. MacAuly (Eds.), *Operant procedures in remedial speech and language training*. Boston: Houghton Mifflin, 1968.

Straughan, J. H., Potter, W. K., & Hamilton, S. H. The behavioral treatment of an elective mute. *Journal of Child Psychology and Psychiatry*, 1965, *6*, 125–230.

Strossen, R. J., Coates, T. J., & Thoresen, C. E. Extending generalizability theory to single subject designs. *Behavior Therapy*, 1979, *10*, 606–614.

Stuart, R. B. *Trick or treatment: How and when psychotherapy fails*. Champaign, Ill.: Research Press, 1970.

Suinn, R. M. *Fundamentals of behavior pathology*. New York: Wiley, 1970.

Sulzer-Azaroff, B., & Mayer, G. R. *Applying behavior-analysis procedures with children and youth*. New York: Holt, Rinehart & Winston, 1977.

Sundberg, N. D. The practice of psychological testing in clinical services in the United States. *American Psychologist*, 1961, *16*, 79–83.

Szasz, T. S. The myth of mental illness. *American Psychologist*, 1960, *15*, 113–118.

Szasz, T. S. *The myth of mental illness*. New York: Harper & Row, 1974.

Tharp, R. G., & Wetzel, R. J. *Behavior modification in the natural environment*. New York: Academic Press, 1969.

Thelen, M. H., Varble, D. L., & Johnson, J. Attitudes of academic clinical psychologists towards projective techniques. *American Psychologist*, 1968, *23*, 517–521.

Thelen, M. H., & Ewing, D. R. Roles, functions, and training in clinical psychology: A survey of academic clinicians. *American Psychologist*, 1970, *25*, 550–554.

Thoresen, C. E. *Let's get intensive: Single case research*. Englewood Cliffs, N.J.: Prentice-Hall, in press.

Thoresen, C. E., & Mahoney, M. *Behavioral self-control*. New York: Holt, Rinehart & Winston, 1974.

Tramer, M. Elektiver mutismus bie kindern. *Zeitschrift fuer Kinderpsychiatrie*, 1934, *1*, 30–35.

Tramer, M. *Lehrbuch der allgemeinen kinderpsychiatrie*. Basel, Switzerland: Schwabe, 1949.

Tramer, M., & Geiger-Martz, O. Zur frage beziehung von elektivem und totalem mutismus des kindersalters. Zeitschrift fuer Kinderpsychiatrie, 1952, *19*, 88–91.

Treidel, L. *Grundriss der sprachstoerungen, deren ursache, verlauf und behandlung*. Berlin: Hirschwald, 1894.

Treuper, J. Ein knabe mit sprechhemmunger auf psychopathischer grundlage Zeitschrift fur Kinder-fehler, 1897, *5*, 138–143.

Tryon, W. W. The test-trait fallacy. *American Psychologist*, 1979, *34*, 402–406.

Ulmann, L. P., & Krasner, L. *A psychological approach to abnormal behavior*. Englewood Cliffs, N.J.: Prentice-Hall, 1969.

Ulmann, L. P., & Krasner, L. *A psychological approach to abnormal behavior*. (2nd ed.). Englewood Cliffs, N.J.: Prentice-Hall, 1975.

Van der Kooy, D., & Webster, C. D. A rapidly effective behavior modification program for an electively mute child. *Journal of Behavior Therapy and Experimental Psychiatry*, 1975, *6*, 149–152.

Von Misch, A. Elektiver mutismus im kindersalter. *Zietschrift fuer Kinderpsychiatrie*, 1952, *19*, 49–87.

Wachtel, P. L. On fact, hunch, and stereotype: A reply to Mischel. *Journal of Abnormal Psychology*, 1973, *82*, 537–540. (a)

Wachtel, P. L. Psychodynamics, behavior therapy, and the implacable experimenter: An inquiry into the consistency of personality. *Journal of Abnormal Psychology*, 1973, *82*, 324–334. (b)

Wade, T. C., & Baker, T. B. Opinions on use of psychological tests: A survey of clinical psychologists. *American Psychologist,* 1977, *32,* 874-882.

Wade, T. C., Baker, T. B., & Hartmann, D. P. Behavior therapists' self-reported views and practices. *The Behavior Therapist,* 1979, *2,* 3-6.

Wade, T. C., Baker, T. B., Morton, T. L., & Baker, L. F. The status of psychological testing in clinical psychology: Relationships between use, test use, and professional activities in orientations. *Journal of Personality Assessment,* 1978, *42,* 3-10.

Wahler, R. G. Some structural aspects of deviant child behavior. *Journal of Applied Behavior Analysis,* 1975, *8,* 27-42.

Wahler, R. G., Berland, R. M., & Coe, T. D. Generalization processes in child behavior change. In B. B. Lahey & A. E. Kazdin (Eds.), *Advances in clinical child psychology* (Vol. 2). New York: Plenum, 1979.

Wallis, H. Zur systematik des mutismus im kindersalter. *Zeitschrift für kinderpsychiatrie,* 1957, *24,* 129-133.

Walton, D., & Black, D. A. The applications of modern learning theory to the treatment of chronic hysterical aphonia. *Journal of Psychosomatic Research,* 1959, *3,* 303-311.

Waternik, J., & Vedder, R. Einige faelle von thymogenem mutismus bei sehr jungen kindern und seine behandlung. *Zeitschrift Kinderforsch, Supplement,* 1936, *45,* 368-369.

Weber, A. Zum elektiven mutisums der kinder. *Zeitschrift fuer Kinderpsychiatrie,* 1950, *17,* 1-15.

Weisman, A. D. Silence and psychotherapy. *Psychiatry,* 1955, *18,* 241-260.

Werner, L. S. Treatment of a child with delayed speech. *Journal of Speech Disorders,* 1945, *10,* 329-334.

Werr, J. S., & Quay, H. C. The prevalence of behavior symptoms in younger elementary school children. *American Journal of Orthopsychiatry,* 1971, *41,* 136-143.

Wetzel, R. J., Balch, P., & Kratochwill, T. R. Behavioral counseling: The environment vs. client. In J. D. Noshpitz (Ed.), *Basic handbook of child psychiatry.* New York: Basic Books, 1979.

Wildman, B. G., & Erickson, M. T. Methodological problems in behavioral observation. In J. D. Cone & R. P. Hawkins (Eds.), *Behavioral assessment: New directions in clinical psychology.* New York: Brunner/Mazel, 1978.

Wildman, R. W. II, & Wildman, R. W. The generalization of behavior modification procedures: A review with special emphasis on classroom applications. *Psychology in the Schools,* 1975, *12,* 432-444.

Williamson, D. A., Sanders, S. H., Sewell, W. R., Haney, J. N., & White, D. The behavioral treatment of elective mutism: Two case studies. *Journal of Behavior Therapy and Experimental Psychiatry,* 1977, *8,* 143-149. (a)

Williamson, D. A., Sewell, W. R., Sanders, S. H., Haney, J. N., & White, D. The treatment of reluctant speech using contingency management procedures. *Journal of Behavior Therapy and Experimental Psychiatry,* 1977, *8,* 155-156. (b)

Willmore, L. The role of speech therapy in voice cases. *Journal of Laryngology,* 1959, *73,* 104.

Wilson, G. T. On the much discussed nature of the term "behavior therapy." *Behavior Therapy,* 1978, *9,* 89-98.

Wilson, M. S. Hysterical aphonia. *American Journal of Psychiatry,* 1962, *19,* 80.

Winkelman, N. W. Diagnosis and treatment of hysterical aphonia. *Medical Clinics of North America,* 1937, *21,* 1211-1220.

Wittenborn, J. Symptom patterns in a group of mental hospital patients. *Journal of Consulting Psychology,* 1951, *15,* 290-302.

Wittenborn, J. The behavioral symptoms for certain organic psychoses. *Journal of Counseling Psychology,* 1952, *16,* 104-106.

Wolf, M. M. Social validity: The case for subjective measurement or how applied behavior analysis is finding its heart. *Journal of Applied Behavior Analysis,* 1978, *11,* 203-214.

Wolf, M. M., Risley, T. R., & Mees, H. L. Applications of operant conditioning procedures to the behavior problems of an autistic child. *Behavior Research and Therapy,* 1964, *1,* 305–312.

Wolpe, J. *Psychotherapy by reciprocal inhibition.* Stanford, Calif.: Stanford University Press, 1958.

Wright, H. F. *Recording and analyzing child behavior: With ecological data from an American town.* New York: Harper & Row, 1968.

Wulbert, M., Nyman, B. A., Snow, I., & Owen, Y. The efficacy of stimulus fading and contingency management in the treatment of elective mutism: A case study. *Journal of Applied Behavior Analysis,* 1973, *6,* 435–441.

Yates, A. G. *Behavior therapy.* New York: Wiley, 1970.

Zeligs, M. A. The psychology of silence. *Journal of the American Psychoanalytic Association,* 1961, *9,* 7–43.

Zigler, E., & Phillips, L. Psychiatric diagnosis and symptomatology. *Journal of Abnormal and Social Psychology,* 1961, *63,* 69–75. (a)

Zigler, E., & Phillips, L. Psychiatric diagnosis: A critique. *Journal of Abnormal and Social Psychology,* 1961, *63,* 607–618. (b)

Zimmerman, B. J., & Rosenthal, T. L. Observational learning of rule-governed behavior by children. *Psychological Bulletin,* 1974, *81,* 29–42.

Zubin, J. Classification of the behavior disorders. In P. R. Farnsworth, O. McNemar, & Q. McNeman (Eds.), *Annual review of psychology.* Palo Alto, Calif.: Annual Reviews, 1967.

Zubin, J. But is it good for science? *Clinical Psychologist,* 1978, *31,* 1.

Printed and bound by CPI Group (UK) Ltd, Croydon, CR0 4YY

22/10/2024

01777615-0013

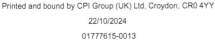

# Author Index

# Subject Index